BREAST CANCER TREATMENT OPTIONS

BREAST CANCER TREATMENT OPTIONS

ROBERT P. LENK

Nova Science Publishers, Inc.
Commack, New York

Editorial Production: Susan Boriotti
Office Manager: Annette Hellinger
Graphics: Frank Grucci and John T'Lustachowski
Information Editor: Tatiana Shohov
Book Production: Donna Dennis, Patrick Davin, Christine Mathosian, Tammy Sauter and Diane Sharp
Circulation: Maryanne Schmidt
Marketing/Sales: Cathy DeGregory

Library of Congress Cataloging-in-Publication Data available upon request

ISBN / 1-56072-396-3

Copyright © 1999 by Robert P. Lenk
       Nova Science Publishers, Inc.
       6080 Jericho Turnpike, Suite 207
       Commack, New York 11725
       Tele. 516-499-3103   Fax 516-499-3146
       e-mail: Novascience@earthlink.net
       e-mail: Novascil@aol.com
       Web Site: http://www.nexusworld.com/nova

Printed in the United States of America

DEDICATION

This work is dedicated to those who struggle so hard to fight cancer:

To the supportive groups of nurses, counselors and staff, who humanize the treament process.

To the physicians, who challenge the odds.

To the researchers who design tools to fight this complex disease.

But most of all, to the patients whose courage inspires us all.

CONTENTS

1

PURPOSE

This guide is written assuming you have been diagnosed as having cancer of the breast. You may have heard that this happens to one in nine women, but no one can be prepared for the shock that follows those ominous words.

The range of emotions that follow diagnosis can run anywhere from sickening fear to anger and denial. Breast cancer is especially devastating because, even though it can often be cured, the prospect of disfigurement from surgery seems unbearable.

At some point in your reaction, you are going to decide to fight back. To do this, you need to know more about the disease, options for treatment, and management of the social aspects of cancer. You must restore control over your body, and make yourself a more effective partner with your physician as you work together to bring you back to health.

The purpose is to help you understand what we know about this disease and the treatment options. There often is no best way to treat cancer, and any information regarding diagnosis or treatment is intended to improve your understanding of the available options. This book is not a substitute for professional medical advice.

Events following the diagnosis of cancer come at a dizzying pace because we know that early and aggressive intervention gives the best chance of curing you, while waiting can be fatal. Too often, physicians fall in the rut of treating the patient as a passive vessel to receive prescribed treatments. They need to be reminded they are treating you, not your tumor.

Most patients feel they've been swept onto an escalator where everyone seems to be requiring critical decisions without giving them a chance to recover from the crushing psychological blow of the diagnosis.

Unfortunately, this can't be helped. Often, there isn't enough time to get answers to all the questions you want to ask your doctor. Everyone's busy, and it's convenient to persuade you that you can't possibly learn enough, so you had better just follow what you're told. This book will help you understand what's going on, so you can contribute to deciding what's best for you.

You can take back the initiative. Physicians sometimes ignore the fact that your participation is critical to the success of your treatment. Too often patients feel they have no more control over events than a leaf in an autumn gust.

This struggle is about your body and your life. You need to assert your rôle as a partner with your physician. To do this, you need information to empower you to help map out a strategy for your treatment.

More importantly, you need to reassert control over your body. The initiative to fight back must come from within you. You need to understand the battle raging inside you, so your desire to prevail can potentiate your therapy, and help cure you. Cancer is born of and propagates chaos, but you can restore order by learning and fighting back.

There is a lot of new vocabulary that easily becomes confusing. To help, there is a glossary at the end; key words underlined in the text are fully explained in sections elsewhere in the book, which you can find in the Table of Contents.

2

Basic Questions

What is Cancer?

Cancer is not really one disease, but a group of diseases whose root cause is chaotic cell growth. The term: "growth" may be a little confusing, since cells in a tissue can grow either by getting bigger or by multiplying in number (proliferating). We use "growth" to mean the latter.

The important thing to understand is that it started because just one of your normal cells became deranged, and its descendants are multiplying to the point they threaten your health. It is not a disease where eliminating some foreign organism ends the disease. To cure cancer every last mutant cell has to be removed or killed. If this is not done even one surviving cancer cell will restart the process.

Removal by surgery is the easiest and most complete treatment if it can be used. However, if the cancer has spread or cannot be physically removed for one reason or another it will be necessary to treat it with some combination of surgery, radiation, hormone and chemotherapy to kill the malignant cells.

More than half of those who have breast cancer can be treated by surgery alone. Those who require chemotherapy should understand that any treatment that is directed to kill cancer cells is going to be toxic for some healthy cells, too, because they are so closely related. The healthy cells that are most susceptible are the ones closest in appearance to the tumor cells.

This balancing act: killing the malignant cells while sparing the healthy ones, is the challenge you are facing. There are some things you can do to help shift the balance in favor of protecting your body and these are explained in the section on Managing Side Effects.

Nothing happens in your body in isolation. Each and every cell is part of a complex interconnected system. What goes on in one place affects what goes on in other tissues as well. This rich symphony of signaling becomes unbalanced by cancer and its therapy.

But there is also a metaphysical factor we do not understand about wellness. Reach inside yourself to feel the struggle within. Enrich your body's defenses with diet, meditation, and faith. These intangible forces will help you regain the initiative. When you assert control, your confidence and determination will maximize the impact of your therapy.

WHAT CAUSES CANCER?

We know that the single cell which produced the tumor did so because of some changes (mutations) in its genetic material, but we can only guess what caused the *mutations*. Normally, for a <u>malignancy</u> to develop, not one, but several genetic changes must take place. In some families people are born with one of the mutations already present. These people are more likely to develop cancer at some time in their life.

In your body, millions of cells are manipulating their DNA every day. When you think about the number it is not surprising that mutations happen quite often. Usually these mistakes are corrected by a DNA repair system. Each cell contains a factory of enzymes whose sole function is fixing mistakes that happen during DNA manipulation.

We can study these processes in the laboratory, but in our bodies, which are infinitely more complicated, we can only guess what factors determine how genetic errors become permament. We believe it is some combination of happenstance and environmental conditions that either increase the frequency of mutations or hamper the repair machinery.

There are factors that go together with cancer so often that we suspect there is a link, like lung cancer and smoking. But there are many cases of lung cancer in people who have never smoked. <u>Statistical analysis</u> is used to measure whether there is likely a link between some environmental condition and cancer.

Our understanding of the causes of breast cancer is even more confused than it is for lung cancer. You often hear in the news about a study of possible dietary influences, or various other exposures that may be factors. Identifying these factors is controversial, sometimes even contradictory. We hope these kinds of studies will someday help us change our environment to make it safer, but we are only beginning to learn how to handle this kind of information.

In theory you should look at the sum of all the exposures over a lifetime, any one of which could have been responsible. We do know that one in nine women will develop breast cancer at some time in their life. Looking at the characteristics of women who develop breast cancer, statistical analysis has shown us some ways of grouping people to find those who have a higher than normal rate of developing cancer.

These groups are described as having a higher than average risk, but most women in high risk groups do not develop cancer. That said, statistics tell us that women whose firstborn came after age 30 are more likely to develop breast cancer. Women who started menstruating early or who go through menopause late also have a higher risk. Excess alcohol or fat consumption may also increase the chances of developing breast cancer.

If cancer comes into your life it may be comforting or useful to reason why. The bottom line is that it is nothing you did, nor could you have prevented it. While there have been many studies of various risk factors, there are few black and white answers.

Mostly this is because we just don't know enough about the disease to put all the pieces of information together in a coherent picture.

WHICH CELL BECOMES MALIGNANT?

It varies. Breast cancer is usually the result of a change in one of the cells of the breast, as you would expect. But there are many different kinds of cell in the breast. As part of the diagnosis, your doctor took a biopsy to have a specialist examine the type of cell in the microscope. This is called histological typing.

Nearly all breast cancer cells are adenocarcinomas. This means the cells have matured enough to be recognizable as cells which are part of the glands in the breast which secrete milk.

The histology also tells us whether the tumor came from cells in the ducts of the secretory gland, or the cells in the lobule of the gland. Three out of four breast cancer patients have ductal cell carcinoma.

Another important analysis of the cells tells whether the hormone estrogen can bind to them or not. These are termed estrogen receptor positive (ER+). Mature glandular cells in the breast have receptors that specifically recognize the hormones estrogen and progesterone.

Hormones like estrogen are messengers, sent from one part of your body to tell other cells what is going on so they can act appropriately. In the case of estrogen, it is produced in your ovaries to signal the stage of your menstrual cycle and whether you are pregnant or not. Estrogen signals the cells in the breast to grow and prepare to produce milk as part of the menstrual cycle. Thus estrogen siganlling is an important part of the normal life cycle of these cells and is used as the basis for hormone therapy, as you will learn shortly.

Just under half of women who develop breast cancer before menopause have ER+ cells, while more than 60% of post-menopausal women have ER+ cells.

Histological typing also tells your doctor whether the cells are growing aggressively or not. This is determined with a variety of techniques designed to measure what fraction of the cells are in mitosis, S phase and G2 phase. These are phases of the Cell Cycle.

Rarer types of cells that form tumors in the breast include skin cells (squamous cell carcinoma), connective tissue cells (sarcoma), and sweat gland cells.

WHAT IS GOING TO HAPPEN?

This critical question is difficult to answer generally. The outcome depends on your specific disease. Factors that affect the outcome include the cell type, the size of the tumor, whether it has spread and where, your age and other health problems that may complicate treatment.

There has been much progress in the last ten years in improving the chances of curing breast cancer, but the prudent course is to prepare for the worst, while expecting the best outcome.

It is important to remember that probabilities are only useful in predicting what will happen to a large number of people and are powerless to forecast what will happen to any individual. It's a lot like predicting coin tosses. We know that if you toss a coin many times, the number of heads will be about the same as the number of tails. However, we cannot say whether the next toss will be a head or a tail. Every patient is unique, and it doesn't matter whether you are the one in three or the one in one hundred; what matters is your specific case.

Another important point is that information about survival only takes into account cases that happened some time ago. Survival is usually measured as how many patients are alive five years after their treatment. If a new way of treating the disease improves the survival of everyone using it, the results will not show up in these survival tables for at least another five years[1].

That said, the statistics are that 186,000 new cases of breast cancer were discovered in 1996 in the US. Overall, nine out of ten women will survive five years or more, based on past history.

3

HOW SERIOUS IS IT?

TYPES OF BREAST CANCER

Most lumps discovered in the breast are harmless. They may be deposits of fat, cysts, or dense clusters of fibroblasts. The latter are specialized cells found in nearly every organ of the body who make the webs of structural fibers that strengthen and shape organs. Masses of fibrous tissue are often called fibroids. They are benign and are composed of different cell types than those that cause malignancies; they cannot become cancer. However, they frequently cause a lot of anxiety, and present a danger because it is difficult to distinguish them from malignant tumors without further testing. Sometimes a malignant tumor is ignored because we assume it's a fibroid.

Inside a breast is an interconnected network of vessels designed to produce milk when called for. There are also fatty deposits, nerves, lymphatics, and a network of fibrous connective tissue that molds and shapes the breast mound. The tubules that channel the milk are called ducts, and the milk producing vessels are called lobules. Epithelial cells make up the lining of both the lobules and the ducts. The latter are the cells that can become malignant and form a tumor. Breast epithelial cells undergo monthly changes as part of the menstrual cycle. Every month these cells begin to grow, multiply and prepare the machinery for milk production, in anticipation of a pregnancy. In the absence of a pregnancy, these cells cease preparation and regress to the normal size.

It is important for you and your physicians to learn as much as possible about the type of tumor you have to decide on the best course of treatment.

Breast cancer is broadly divided into two categories, localized (also called *in situ*) and invasive tumors.

In situ tumors have not penetrated the lining of the ducts or lobules. In the microscope they appear different from normal cells, forming a chaotic, irregular clump (called a dysplasia). They are not malignant, but may become so in time. When found in the ducts of the breast, localized tumors are usually removed before that can happen.

Invasive tumors are those that have begun to infiltrate the surrounding tissues. Often they spread through the milk ducts. Ductal cell carcinomas are the most common form of breast cancer, and the type we have most success treating.

Lobular tumors, which account for about 10% of breast cancers, don't feel like lumps, but like a thickening of the breast tissue. Usually lobular tumors are present in both breasts by the time they are discovered and have often spread other places as well.

Inflammatory breast cancer is a rare type of invasive cancer that often feels like an infection, i.e. there is an area that is swollen, red and hot. These symptoms arise because the tumor has penetrated the local lymphatics and has provoked a response similar to the inflammation you get from a local infection. Sometimes inflammatory breast cancer causes a swelling of the lymphatics within the breast, which makes the skin dimple, like an orange rind.

Paget's disease is a rare type of cancer associated with the nipple. It causes local bleeding, scaling, itching or burning.

Medullary carcinoma is formed from cells of the skin, and has a distinctive appearance from tubular carcinoma in biopsies.

Mucinus carcinoma is an uncommon glandular tumor that produces a sticky secretion.

EVALUATING BREAST CANCER

Staging is an evaluation of the severity of a patient's disease. It is convenient to classify four stages, although you will see that these four stages are broken up into smaller subgroups as well. We use the staging system to pool individuals into groups whose disease is more or less equivalent, and to evaluate the risks and recommended therapies appropriate to how serious the disease is.

The diagnostic tools that help determine the staging include tools for visualizing the tumor, such as mammograms (and other x-rays), ultrasound, MRI and the CT (also call CAT) scan.

Sometimes, breast cancer spreads from the primary site and forms secondary tumors (called metastases). Often it goes first to the lymphatics. These include the axillary nodes (located in the armpit), clavicular nodes (located above and below the collar bone) and the cervical lymph nodes (neck). In some cases, your doctor can feel lumps in these lymph nodes, but he may need to remove them and have a pathologist examine the tissues for tumors too small to feel.

Your Doctor may also test to see if the cancer has spread to other organs (metastasized). The techniques used are bone scans (which use 99Tc to detect tumors in the bone), CT (computerized tomography, a kind of three dimensional x-ray) or MRI (magnetic resonance imaging) scans to visualize possible tumors. If present, metastases are usually found in the skin, lung, brain and liver. You should know that these tests cannot see tiny tumors in these sites. Unfortunately, just because metastases haven't been seen does not mean there are none present.

The classification system changes as we learn more about breast cancer, and there are differences of opinion over how much weight to put on the various factors used in classifying which stage a patient falls into. The tables following give the criteria used most often.

Staging Criteria for Breast Cancer

Stage	Tumor Size	Lymph Node Involvement	Distant Metastasis
0	*in situ*	N0 (none)	-
I	T1	N0	-
IIa	T0	N1	-
	T1	N1	-
	T2	N0	-
IIb	T2	N1	-
	T3	N0	-
IIIa	T0	N2	-
	T1, T2	N2	
	T3	N1, N2	-
IIIb	Any	N3	-
	T4	Any	-
IV	Any	Any	Yes

One important category for grouping is the size of the primary tumor. The following table explains how tumor sizes are categorized.

Tumor Size Classification

T0	No evidence of tumor
T1	Largest diameter is 2 cm or less
T2	Largest diameter between 2 and 5 cm
T3	Largest diameter over 5 cm
T4	Tumor invades chest wall or skin

Classification of Lymph Node Involvement

The degree of lymph node involvement is also important in evaluating how to treat you. Usually, spreading (metastasizing) cells form tumors in the lymph nodes, which can sometimes be detected by feeling them (called palpation). The following table shows one way of evaluating how to categorize different stages of node involvement.

Nodal Categories

N0	No malignant cells detected
N1	Axillary nodes (those in the armpit) on the same side as the tumor (ipsilateral) are enlarged but still can be moved around
N2	Axillary nodes are enlarged and are no longer movable because they have become attached to each other or other structures
N3	Tumor has invaded the mammary lymph nodes.
N4	Superclavicular lymph nodes involved (Those above the collar bone)

Other Methods for Classifying Tumors

Some physicians use a simpler system to classify patients. They use the above system for Stage 0, I and IV, but characterize patients with lymph node involvement solely on how many nodes are found to contain malignant cells when examined. They might classify patients with more than 10 lymph nodes as one group, 4 to 10 as another, and less than 4 as a third group.

While most types of breast cancer are caused by malignant growth of the epithelial cells of the gland, these cancer cells are not all the same. We are now developing tools that help us characterize specific features of the different cell types, to distinguish different types of breast cancer and tailor treatment for each type. The cell properties that are most generally accepted are listed here, while the more experimental methods are described later in the section entitled "Genetic Probes."

Mitotic Index

The proportion of cells in the different phases of the <u>cell cycle</u> tells your doctor how many of the cells in the tumor are multiplying. There are tests that determine how many cells are in M, S and G2 phase. If the tumor is growing slowly, many more cells will be in G1 phase, but if all the cells are cycling, the fraction of cells in the M and S phases will be higher. Treatment options for a slowly growing tumor are different from those for an aggressive tumor.

Estrogen Receptors

A distinction that has important consequences is whether you have gone through menopause or not. This is significant because post menopausal women are no longer producing estrogen, a signal molecule that communicates with many cells, including those of the breast.

Careful examination of the malignant cells that produced the tumor will reveal whether or not the cells are equipped with the growth signal receptor on their surface that binds estrogen. Just under half the tumors in premenopausal women are estrogen receptor positive (ER+). For postmenopausal women the percentage is higher (between 60 and 70%). If the cells have estrogen receptors they usually will stop growing when exposed to hormone therapy with drugs like Tamoxifen.

4

OVERVIEW OF TREATMENT OPTIONS

STAGE 0, I AND II

Fortunately, most women diagnosed with breast cancer have Stage 0 and I tumors. If you are one of these consider yourself extremely fortunate, and give credit to yourself and those who helped find it. Early stage disease is nearly always curable. These tumors can be removed surgically by either a lumpectomy or removal of the entire breast. Often surgery includes the *lymph* nodes under the arm which are examined to make sure the cancer hasn't spread. More than 9 out of 10 women with stage I disease will survive at least five years[2].

Treatment of Stage II disease is nearly as effective. 7 out of 10 women will survive 5 years or more. The survival figures are lower due to imperfections in our ability to detect disease that has spread. Stage II disease is treated successfully with surgery and/or radiotherapy, often followed with hormone therapy.

Chemotherapy is used to kill cells that have spread beyond the local area, but it is a dangerous weapon. There is a risk that the drugs used in chemotherapy will cause you health problems later on, even induce another cancer. For this reason, Stage II disease is not usually treated with chemotherapy after the primary treatment.

Often radiotherapy is employed after the surgery to kill any cells in the vicinity of the primary tumor that escaped resection. The decision whether to treat with radiotherapy depends on how confident your doctor is the tumor can be removed by surgery. If there is any evidence the tumor has invaded the chest muscles, for example, radiation would probably be used.

Radiation works by causing lethal genetic damage in the bombarded cells. Some cells on the fringe of the irradiated area may also receive insults that cause increased genetic damage. This is a controversial subject, but some physicians believe radiation should not be used because it can lead to the development of other cancers. Others feel the risk is insignificant compared to the risk of you dying from your cancer. A factor in deciding whether to use radiation or not is your age. The younger you are the greater the chances that a radiation induced mutation can transform into a malignancy ten years from now.

You and your physician must discuss your situation and judge whether the risk of health problems later are too high compared to the risk that your cancer will already have spread by the time it is treated. This is a critical question, and you need to satisfy yourself that it has been considered carefully.

DETECTION OF METASTASES

We do know the overall statistics about undetected metastases. About one in four women who had no detectable node involvement will later develop disease because some cells had spread before treatment.

Three out of four women who had tumors in their axillary lymph nodes will relapse because some cells had already spread beyond the local area and caused new tumors.

STAGE III AND IV

Treatment of late stage disease (IIIa, IIIb and IV) involves difficult decisions. When the nodal status is 2 or 3, or there are distant metastases, we must depend on chemotherapy to kill all the pockets of cells away from the primary site. While the statistics don't include new breakthroughs in treatment, you should know this happens less often than we would like. While there are thousands of cases where late stage disease has been treated successfully, less than half of women with Stage III disease will be alive in five years, if events follow historical trends. The odds are worse with Stage IV.

You and your doctors must evaluate your particular disease and examine the different options to decide the best way to treat your breast cancer. New drugs, new ways of combining drugs with surgery and/or radiation may be considered in determining what is best for you.

Today, the trend is to treat first with <u>combination chemotherapy</u>, and see how well the cancer responds. Often this is all that is needed. If it comes back, your options are to undergo a similar treatment or try some aggressive new technique, such as high dose therapy with <u>growth factor support</u>.

There are a number of experimental approaches that have not been around long enough to be considered proven. You need to have a realistic appreciation of the severity of your disease to decide whether these make sense for you. Approach the decision knowledgeably, and assert your opinions with your physician, so you can become a partner in the strategy for managing your disease.

If there is a high probability that your disease can be managed with known therapies, you may be better off electing a proven treatment. To make this decision you need to know the number of patients that have been evaluated with this therapy, and the outcome. It would be especially useful to know how many patients there were in the study(s) who had a similar stage disease to yours, and how they fared.

On the other hand, if your disease is more advanced you may want to try an experimental approach. Your options include neoadjuvant therapy, or a combination of drugs that includes one of the new agents, or a new technique in combined modality therapy. It is a tough choice, best made by learning as much as you can. If these options are not available with your physician, find another doctor. This is not a time to let convenience dictate your choices.

OTHER TYPES OF BREAST CANCER

Rarer forms of the disease, such as mucinus or inflammatory breast cancer, don't respond to standard treatment, and you and your physician should consider experimental therapy for these settings.

WHAT HAPPENS IN TREATMENT?

Cancer is caused by your own cells becoming unable to regulate their rate of growth due to mutations in the DNA of a cell which passed the change on to its daughters. Treatment requires eliminating each one of the offspring of these cells.

Surgery

Surgical resection (mastectomy) is the most effective treatment. If no tumor cells are left behind, surgery will cure you of the disease. However, if even one cell escaped, either because it had broken off the primary tumor and landed in a secondary site, or removal of the tumor was incomplete, then the whole process will begin again. The problem for the surgeon is that he cannot see individual cells, so he must remove all the tissue that could contain malignant cells.

The more confined the tumor, the more likely the surgeon will be able to resect all the tumor cells. Unfortunately, some patients with breast cancer have tumors which cannot be completely removed, and some additional treatment must be used to kill those cells that are outside the part the surgeon removes.

Lumpectomy

One of the significant advances we have made in the last decade is due to the systematic analysis by the NSABP comparing radical mastectomy with local removal (lumpectomy) plus radiation therapy in Stage I and II breast cancer. This large trial showed that, for certain tumors, it is not necessary to perform radical surgery, and many women have been spared the psychological blow of disfigurement due to this work.

Recently media reports suggested there was some question as to the validity of these results. The disclosures revealed inconsistencies in the way the data was collected from one of the many hospitals participating in the study. Whatever the motive behind these public revelations, they destroyed the reputation of the head of the NSABP and caused much alarm.

You should know that the conclusions of this study were in no way affected by these discrepancies. The study was designed so that no single site could bias the outcome, and the results were the same whether the data from the suspect hospital were included or not. Since then other, independent groups[3],[4] have made similar comparisons, and come to the same conclusion.

This is not to say that all cases of breast cancer can be treated with a lumpectomy. You and your surgeon will evaluate whether this can be applied to your condition.

Radiation

Radiation is used when the chances are good that surgery alone will not remove every last tumor cell. If the cancer has spread too far into the adjoining tissues, or the surgeon believes some cells might escape, then radiation may be used by itself or in combination with surgical resection. Often, if your physicians suspect the cancer has spread beyond the local area, radiation may be used in concert with chemotherapy to treat the disease.

What is it?

Radiotherapy uses ionizing radiation to kill cells exposed to the field. For radiotherapy, the source of radiation can be x-rays, electron beams or radioactive isotopes.

Ionizing radiation is a form of electromagnetic radiation, like light, microwaves or radio waves. It is a high energy radiation that zaps the molecules in the field of radiation, ionizing them. Ionized molecules are especially lethal to growing cells. Some cells are killed immediately by ionization, but most die because the DNA has been damaged, which blocks replication, so they can't continue the <u>cell cycle</u>.

External Radiation

There are different sources for the x-rays that can be used in radiotherapy, and each has different properties.

Low energy x-rays are emitted by orthovoltage machines. The x-rays given off have energy levels of about 300,000 Volts (300 kV). Such x-rays do not penetrate very deeply inside tissues, so they are used mostly for treating skin cancer.

High energy (over 1,000 kV) x-rays are given off by Megavoltage machines. Another source of 1,000 kV radiation is from the radioactive substance Cobalt 60 that is housed in a lead container with a removable cover. Either of these sources produces radiation that can penetrate up to 2 inches beneath the surface of the skin.

Linear Accelerators produce either electron beams or x-rays or a mixed beam at energy levels between 4,000 and 35,000 kV (4,000,000 to 35,000,000 Volts). This expensive machine offers a lot of versatility, since the level of penetration of the electron beam can be controlled by how much energy is used to energize the beam.

The radiotherapist (sometimes called a radiation oncologist) plans the field of treatment very carefully to maximize the exposure to the malignant tissue and minimize damage to healthy organs. The first decision is how to line up the x-ray beam such that it will avoid sensitive areas and fully encompass the tumor region. The beam path is called the "radiation port." Sometimes special screens will be used to block the x-rays from hitting vital tissues. Planning the radiation port often involves other experts, such as a dosimetrist and/or a clinical physicist.

Setting up the radiation port and appropriate screens may involve a "dress rehearsal" with a simulator. Again, the purpose is to plan the exposure to minimize damage to healthy, vital tissues, and make sure the entire tumor area is receiving the full treatment.

Sometimes the radiation will be given during surgery so the radiotherapist can access the area during its exposure for surgery.

The dose of radiotherapy is measured in centiGrays (cGy[5]). Different tissues have different sensitivities. Breasts can tolerate 2,000 cGy. This means that the radiation dose to the entire breast cannot exceed that. The portion of the breast encompassing the tumor, of course, should be higher.

Once the Radiotherapist has determined the dose necessary to kill the tumor, (s)he will decide how to deliver it. It has been proven that dividing the dose over 10 to 20 treatments (fractions) is less harmful to the healthy tissues without losing anti-tumor activity. Therefore radiotherapy is usually given in multiple doses, spread out over a few weeks.

SIDE EFFECTS

A lot depends on which tissues in the radiation field are affected, so it is difficult to generalize. The following apply to chest irradiation.

Fatigue is the most commonly experienced side effect from radiation therapy, often accompanied by a general uncomfortable feeling, or uneasiness (malaise). The severity of this varies from almost none to very disturbing. It will go away after a while, but can last several weeks.

Nausea and vomiting are unusual after radiotherapy, unless the upper abdomen is included in the field.

Skin toxicity. With the use of multiple ports and high energy beams the affect on the skin is not as bad as it was in the past. Nevertheless, radiotherapy has been compared to severe sunburn (or even barbecue). Redness (erythema) similar to sunburn can occur, which peels in time. It should disappear after a week or two. Increased pigmentation can occur a while after therapy, especially in darker skinned individuals.

Esophageal damage. Chest x-rays often include the tube connecting your mouth to the stomach (esophagus) in the field, which can produce symptoms like heartburn. It is due to irritation of the lining of the esophagus by the radiation. It will go away, and antacids will help treat the symptoms.

Hormone Therapy

Many breast cancer cells carry estrogen receptors (termed ER+), and grow when estrogen is present. Drugs like Tamoxifen and Megesterol are man-made compounds designed to bind to the estrogen receptor, so that the estrogen signal never gets heard. Hormone therapy does not kill tumor cells, but shuts them off, so to speak, so they no longer grow in response to estrogen. As a result, the number of tumor cells is reduced after hormone therapy. The drugs are given daily for two or more years after treatment to keep any tumor cells in perpetual limbo.

Clinical trials have shown us that ER+ women who take Tamoxifen following primary therapy have a better chance of surviving 5 years than those who don't. We don't yet know when it is safe to discontinue hormone therapy.

In principal, the cells should start growing again when you discontinue Tamoxifen, but something seems to happen to eliminate them in many patients. We know this indirectly, by studying survival rates. Since more women survive after Tamoxifen is discontinued, we conclude that something has happened to neutralize or eliminate the cells that were malignant but stopped growing due to the hormone therapy.

Generally, we believe it is best to continue Tamoxifen at least two years. After that, it is an individual question, involving how bad the side effects are, and other factors that will help make the decision when, if ever, to stop. There are some new drugs, designed to be better than Tamoxifen, but we don't yet have as much information about how well they work and their side effects.

Chemotherapy

Chemotherapy is based on the idea of circulating highly poisonous chemicals in the body; poisons that will kill tumor cells but have less effect on normal cells.

Tumor cells differ from most of the body's cells because they are almost always reproducing. Most mature cells have stopped multiplying, so drugs that attack the machinery involved in duplication will be more likely to kill tumor cells. Unfortunately there are some normal cells that also multiply rapidly, like the cells lining the stomach and intestines, or the <u>stem cells</u> producing new blood cells. Such cells become targets as well, and serious side effects result from their being killed by chemotherapy.

Chemotherapy is the only weapon that can kill cells that have spread to other organs (metastasized), and it is used whenever your doctor suspects that metastases are present. Remember that distant tumors are only detected when they have become quite large, and there is a real risk that there are tiny colonies (micrometastases) present that haven't grown enough to be detected yet.

We do not have the ability to selectively treat only tumor cells. Some normal cells are affected as well, and that is what causes the toxic side effects of chemotherapy. Each drug and combination of drugs has its own toxicity profile, which are listed in the section *Drugs used in Chemotherapy.*

You and your physician must evaluate whether the chances of removing all of the tumor cells by surgery or radiation is high and the potential benefits from chemotherapy are worth the side effects.

The choice of what drug or combination of drugs to use depends on the cell the tumor came from. Some kinds of tumors are naturally resistant to certain drugs, either because the drug just doesn't kill them or it doesn't flow to the tumor site in high enough concentrations to kill the cells. This information is determined by <u>clinical trials</u> as new drugs are tested in different types of cancer.

With almost all anti-cancer drugs, we believe that the more drug we give, the better the chance of killing the cells responsible for causing tumors. When new medicines or tricks become available to control the side effects, doctors tend to use this as an opportunity to increase the amount of drug, trying to kill a few thousand more tumor cells and increase your chances of eliminating the disease from your body.

Chemotherapy will make you so sick you will probably wonder which is worse. It is little consolation that the sicker you are, the better your chances of curing your disease.

Administration often involves intravenous infusion of one or more drugs. This can be done in the hospital or at home. Some drugs, like the anthracyclines and mitomycin, are very destructive to local tissues should the needle accidentally escape the vein during infusion. To avoid this hazard, the person administering the drug will insert a long, thin catheter up the vein so the drug actually enters the bloodstream well away from the point of insertion. This catheter may be left in place until your treatment is finished.

Chemotherapy is both physically and emotionally traumatic. Many treatment centers offer special guidance and counseling services to help you. Whether you respond best to counseling or meditation or faith, you should find a way to reach inside yourself for the strength to approach it with calmness. Those who transcend their anxieties have less severe side effects and a better overall experience.

Combination Chemotherapy

Chemotherapy is usually given as a combination of two or more drugs, each of which has its individual strengths and weaknesses. In combination, these "cocktails" attack cancer cells on multiple levels at once, which makes them more effective.

Many "cocktails" include a nitrogen mustard alkylating agent, such as Cyclophosphamide or Ifosfamide. Many also include an anthracycline, such as Doxorubicin, Mitoxantrone or Epirubicin. Other drugs that are often used are 5-Fluorouracil, Methotrexate, one of the vinca alkaloids, and Mitomycin C.

As you can see in the appendix, there are many drugs, and many more combinations than given here. Your doctor may have good reasons for using a different recipe.

The following are the most widely used cocktails for breast cancer therapy. Different treatment centers may adapt one of these by varying the <u>dose</u> slightly, and doses are often adjusted for individual patients. The doses and schedules presented here are to illustrate the variety of combinations and dosing schedules possible. Do not be concerned if yours is not exactly like one of these. On the other hand, it doesn't hurt to ask, and it will help you assert your position as a partner.

Selected Combination Recipes

Acronym	Drug	Dose	Day of Treatment
AC	Doxorubicin	45 mg/M^2 *i.v.*	1
	Cyclophosphamide	500 mg/M^2 *i.v.*	1
		Repeat	every 21 days
CA	Cyclophosphamide	200 mg/M^2 *oral*	1 through 14
	Doxorubicin	40 mg/M^2 *i.v.*	1
		Repeat	every 21-28 days
CAF	Cyclophosphamide	100 mg/M^2 *oral*	1 - 14
	Doxorubicin	30 mg/M^2 *i.v.*	1, 8
	5-Fluorouracil	400 - 500 mg/M^2 *i.v.*	1, 8
		Repeat	every 28 days
CFM	Cyclophosphamide	500 mg/M^2 *i.v.*	1
	5-Fluorouracil	500 mg/M^2 *i.v.*	1
	Mitoxantrone	10 mg/M^2 *i.v.*	1
		Repeat	every 21 days

Table (Continued)

CFPT	Cyclophosphamide	150 mg/M^2 i.v.	1 - 5
	5-Fluorouracil	300 mg/M^2 i.v.	1 - 5
	Prednisone	10 mg oral (3X)	1 - 7
	Tamoxifen	10 mg oral (2X)	every day
		Repeat	every 6 weeks
CMF	Cyclophosphamide	100 mg/M^2 oral or 400 - 600 mg/M^2 i.v.	1 - 14 1
	Methotrexate	40 - 60 mg/M^2 i.v.	1, 8
	5-Fluorouracil	400 - 600 mg/M^2 i.v.	1, 8
		Repeat	every 28 days
CMFP	Cyclophosphamide	100 mg/M^2 oral	1 - 14
	Methotrexate	60 mg/M^2 i.v.	1, 8
	5-Fluorouracil	700 mg/M^2 i.v.	1, 8
	Prednisone	40 mg oral	1 - 14
		Repeat	every 28 days
CMFVP	Cyclophosphamide	2 - 2.5 mg/kg oral	daily for 9 mos.
	Methotrexate	0.7 mg/kg i.v.	weekly for 8 wks then
	5-Fluorouracil	12 mg/kg i.v.	weekly for 7 mos
	Vincristine	0.035 mg/kg i.v.	weekly for 5 wks then
	Prednisone	0.75 mg/kg oral	daily for 10 d. then
CMFVP	Cyclophosphamide	400 mg/M^2 i.v.	1
	Methotrexate	30 mg/M^2 i.v.	1, 8
	5-Fluorouracil	400 mg/M^2 i.v.	1, 8
	Vincristine	1 mg i.v.	1, 8
	Prednisone	20 mg oral (4X)	1 - 7
		Repeat	every 28 days

Table (Continued)

CMFVP	Cyclophosphamide	60 mg/M^2 oral	daily for 1 yr.
	Methotrexate	15 mg/M^2 i.v.	weekly for 1 yr.
	5-Fluorouracil	300 mg/M^2 i.v.	weekly for 1 yr.
	Vincristine	0.625 mg/M^2 i.v.	weekly for 10 wks.
	Prednisone	30 mg/M^2 oral	d1 - 14, then
		20 mg/M^2 oral	d 14 - 28, then
		10 mg/M^2 oral	d 29 - 42
FAC	5-Fluorouracil	500 mg/M^2 i.v.	1, 8
	Doxorubicin	50 mg/M2 i.v.	1
	Cyclophosphamide	500 mg/M2 i.v.	1
		Repeat	every 21 days
IMF	Ifosfamide	15 mg/M2 i.v.	1, 8
	Mesna	One fifth the Ifosfamide dose i.v.	Immediately before, 4 and 8 hrs after Ifosfamide dose
	Methotrexate	40 mg/M2 i.v.	1, 8
	5-Fluorouracil	600 mg/M2 i.v.	1, 8
		Repeat	every 28 days
MMM	Mitoxantrone	8 mg/M2 i.v.	1
	Methotrexate	35 mg/M2 i.v.	1
	Mitomycin C	8 mg/M2 i.v.	1 (alternate courses only)
		Repeat	every 21 days
NFL	Mitoxantrone	12 mg/M2 i.v.	1
	Leucovorin	300 mg/M2 i.v.	1 - 3
	5-Fluorouracil	350 mg/M2 i.v.	After Leucovorin
		Repeat	every 21 days
	Mitoxantrone	10 mg/M2 i.v.	1
	Leucovorin	100 mg/M2 i.v.	1 - 3
	5-Fluorouracil	1000 mg/M2/d	After Leucovorin
		Repeat	every 21 days
VATH	Vinblastine	4.5 mg/M2 i.v.	1
	Doxorubicin	45 mg/M2 i.v.	1
	Thiotepa	12 mg/M2 i.v.	1
	Fluoxymesterone	30 mg oral	Daily throughout
		Repeat	every 21 days

Biological Therapy

We know that tumors, sometimes very large ones, can suddenly disappear even if they aren't treated (the term for this is spontaneous remission). We don't see this very often, but the fact that it can happen tells us that the body is capable of mounting a response that eliminates the tumor. Our bodies have the ability to fight tumors through the immune system and the molecules they give off to eliminate malignancies. The modern tools of molecular biology have helped a number of scientists discover the nature of this remission.

Some of the molecules given off by cells of the immune system to kill tumors are: interferons, interleukins, and tumor necrosis factor. These agents are being studied in clinical trials to find the best way to use them or combine them with other agents to eliminate malignancies. So far, we have seen some interesting results, but they haven't replaced conventional chemotherapy except in special settings. This is a new approach to treatment, and we are still learning about the different tools and how to use them.

WHAT HAPPENS AFTER TREATMENT?

Treatment of Stage 1 and 2 breast cancer is usually successful. The tumor is eliminated and you can expect to be free of disease. Of course you can never free yourself of worry, but the chances are good that you are cured. Many patients with advanced disease are likewise cured.

What about the rest? Patients usually respond to their treatment. Responses vary between patients and stages of disease. They range from apparent elimination of the tumor (complete response) to barely detectable changes. A partial response is usually defined as tumor shrinkage of more than 50%.

Many patients with complete responses never have a problem again. However, too often a response, even a complete response, is only temporary, and the cancer returns later (relapses).

The period during which the tumor is apparently gone is called remission. A remission can last anywhere from a few months to more than five years. If you relapse, there is still a good chance that consolidation therapy can induce another remission. Some patients go more than ten years alternating periods of remission and relapse.

Patients in their first relapse can be offered one of the experimental therapies. You may be a candidate for bone marrow transplantation, or you may wish to try an experimental trial. To evaluate whether you should enroll in an experimental procedure, you should learn some more about the nature of your disease. You should also learn about clinical trials, and have a realistic appraisal of the chances for success.

EXPERIMENTAL TRIALS

Over the last few years, many new drugs have become available, as have new ways of using them. These treatments offer many promising choices, although the results have not yet shown up in five year survival tables. If you have late stage disease, you may wish to participate in one of these experimental trials, or learn about these new developments.

Techniques such as bone marrow transplant allow us to increase the intensity of chemotherapy, and there have been some remarkable improvements in survival because higher doses can kill more malignant cells than traditional means.

Neoadjuvant therapy has been promising in certain settings, and there are new ways of administering radiation that may prove more beneficial.

The problem is that most of these have been studied in a fairly small number of patients in clinical trials, and we won't know for years which will work when applied to large numbers of patients. It is nearly impossible for a trained oncologist to know which of the many experimental alternatives will turn out to improve survival, and it is even harder for an untrained person.

Nevertheless, you have a right to know what is being tried experimentally, and this book will try and guide you through the uncertainties.

Access to Information

The information gathered from these experimental trials is published in the scientific literature, but that is not easy to access or understand. Every year there is a large meeting, organized by the American Society of Clinical Oncologists (ASCO)[6], where studies are reported. Educational sessions are sponsored by ASCO, where noted oncologists summarize the information gleaned from ongoing trials. This is really necessary to help doctors sort through the huge amount of data. For example, at the 1995 ASCO meeting, there were 1,811 papers presented, over 200 on breast cancer alone.

Another valuable source of information is available through the National Cancer Institute. The Physician Data Query (PDQ) system is available as an on-line resource for physicians to access the latest information on prevention and treatment, as well as a list of ongoing clinical trials. Patient information is also provided through the NCI Cancer Information Service[7], which provides hard copy publications, an internet connection to the World Wide Web, and telefax services.

CLINICAL TRIALS: COMPARING NEW TREATMENTS

You should understand how we learn whether a given treatment is better or worse than another. The process is a long one and may seem too drawn out. There are many variables in determining how effective a new treatment is, and a system has been devised over the last fifty years that has proven reliable for evaluating these variables. The process for testing proposed new treatments is called clinical trials.

The most important part of the clinical trial is the patient. Everyone, including the FDA, the hospital, and the investigators, is concerned with the risks to patients participating in clinical trials. The advantages to the medical community of clinical trials cannot be underestimated. Without them, patients may be treated, but there is no way to compare one patient's experience with another's, and we would have no scientific analysis to evaluate which therapies to use and how to use them.

Consider the lumpectomy procedure. Without a large scientific trial we never would have been able to make the statement that lumpectomies are safe. Physicians would use the technique or not use it, depending on whether they considered the liability of failure more important than the psychological benefit to their patients, but no one would know which was right.

We are at a similar situation today with growth factor support. Until large scale randomized trials are carried out and evaluated, we won't know whether this new procedure really is beneficial or not. Unfortunately, very few patients are entering these trials.

Informed Consent

Every patient that enters a clinical trial must sign a detailed informed consent prior to enrollment. This document explains the objectives of the trial, the risks of participating, and other options available. The purpose is to insure that those who participate are given the best information available before they make the decision to volunteer for a study.

Study Objectives

A clinical trial is a scientific study designed to ask one or a few very specific questions about an experimental treatment; these are called the study objectives. For a brand new drug, the question is often "How much of this drug can you give before you cause toxicity?" For a drug that is further advanced in studies, it might be "How effective is this drug against breast cancer compared with another?" The objective must be clearly stated before the trial begins, and the study is designed to answer the central question.

The reason for centering on the objectives in advance is to eliminate the confusing data that evolve when a study's objectives fluctuate as data become available. In the past, investigators tended to "wing it," and see what happens. This very often generates data that are incomprehensible, wasting everyone's time and putting patients at risk for no purpose.

It is also important in designing a clinical trial to specify in advance the criteria for how the results will be interpreted.

A patient may be interested in only one result: "Will it cure me?" But "cure" is a difficult term to define, when you think about it. There is no point at which you can stop wondering if the disease may return. We often draw the line at five years. You will frequently see success measured as five year survival in cancer studies (sometimes early results might be expressed as one or two year survival in ongoing trials).

Survival is not a good measure of success early in the process of evaluating a new therapy. It doesn't make sense to wait five years after the last patient is entered into the trial before proceeding to the next step.

In early studies, the criteria for success is often "response," meaning the tumor shrinks. The precise definition for levels of response varies for different types of cancer. Basically, responses are characterized as either: complete (elimination of the tumor), partial (tumor shrunk more than 50%), stable disease (didn't get worse) or none. The exact meaning of each of these terms is defined in the protocol.

A response, even a complete remission, does not necessarily mean that a patient will survive longer. We also follow those patients who showed a response and see how they fare. These data might be described as how many patients are alive after a given period. In the jargon of cancer studies, there are a few commonly used terms: Overall Survival is abbreviated OS, No Evidence of Disease is abbreviated NED, Disease Free Survival is abbreviated DFS.

Another measure of outcome is called "Quality of Life." This is a new concept, and there is a lot of controversy surrounding its use. For one, patients and physicians may have different definitions of how to measure it. Doctors tend to consider longevity as the most important, while patients may consider a combination of longevity and how well they feel. Yet a third bias is the overall cost of various treatment options. This is too complicated a subject to address here, but you should know about it.

Eligibility Criteria

Once the investigators have clearly defined the question they wish to answer, the next decision is to determine the best group of patients in which to answer it. One of the sources of uncertainty is how to group patients as more or less comparable.

This is often done using the staging system described above, but you can appreciate that, no matter how similar the staging, a 70 year old patient faces different problems than a 35 year old. Yet for evaluation purposes, they may be grouped together. Sometimes it is important to place strict limits on the characteristics for eligibility, and other times it is best to leave the criteria as broad as possible.

Number of Patients

Depending on the nature of the trial, it may require as few as twenty or as many as 1,000 patients to get enough information to answer the questions stated in the objective. Statisticians tell us how many patients are needed in two comparative groups to enable us to answer the question with a high degree of certainty. Clearly, it doesn't take many patients to reveal large differences between two groups, but if the differences are subtle, many more patients will be required.

Types of Clinical Trials

The preliminary studies are designed to define how well a drug (or combination of drugs) is tolerated, how it interacts with the body and what the side effects are. These are called Phase I studies, and are usually performed in patients who have failed to respond to the available treatments, but elect to participate in experimental trials.

Phase II trials are generally small (20 to 50 patients) studies. Experimental treatments are not used as front-line therapy if there are other options available that are known to be effective.

Phase II studies of a new drug are usually carried out in patients who are not expected to benefit from other alternatives. This means patients with late stage disease who have relapsed at least once after standard treatment. Unfortunately, it is hard to decide whether a poor response in these patients means that the drug wouldn't work in early stage disease.

Recently, however, a study showed that giving an experimental drug prior to standard therapy did not compromise patients' chances of survival[8]. This approach may change the way we test new agents in the future.

If a drug has shown promising activity it will be tested as a front-line therapy, often in combination with other agents that are known to be effective. Most chemotherapy is administered as a "cocktail" of two or more drugs, so it is important to study how the new agent interacts with other drugs.

Once it has moved to front-line therapy, the drug can be tested in relatively early stage disease, in a narrowly defined subset of patients who are most likely to benefit. If the patients in these small studies do well, the treatment will be studied later in a larger patient population (Phase III).

This approach of focusing in on small groups is done to control the risk. Patients who enroll in studies of experimental cancer treatments are risking their lives. Therefore the testing of a new treatment is done in as few patients as possible.

However, there can be a lot of confusion when the initial studies are positive. Many experimental treatments turn out to be less effective than originally thought when tested in larger trials. As you read through the various experimental trial results, bear in mind this phenomenon.

Another important difference between the early tests and the large trials is that the latter are carried out in several hospitals by many investigators. Whatever the reason, it has been found that when a treatment is tested in many unrelated sites, positive results from Phase II studies tend to look less favorable. This doesn't mean the original investigators were intentionally biasing the results, but there are many subtle nuances that the originators apply that won't be used by other physicians. If these nuances are important for successful outcome, it is necessary to define them in a multi-center trial, where most of the investigators will be strictly following the treatment as specified.

When experimental therapies have passed these initial tests, they are evaluated by one of the oncology groups in definitive trials. There are groups of opinion leaders, such as the Cancer and Leukemia Group B (CALGB), the South Western Oncology Group (SWOG), Eastern Cooperative Oncology Group (ECOG), or the National Surgical Adjuvant Breast and Bowel Project (NSABP) to name only a few. The members pool their resources to address the pressing questions about treatment options in very large, well planned trials that provide definitive answers to the questions they formulate.

It is best to do double blind studies, so that neither the patient nor the physician knows which treatment a patient is getting. This is usually impossible in cancer trials, because drugs are easily identified by color or other physical properties.

One way to minimize bias in large clinical trials is to randomize patients to different treatments. A study is usually designed to compare a group of patients who receive the best known treatment with one or more groups who receive alternative treatments.

Randomized means that patients who are eligible for the study are selected at random for one or the other treatment. This prevents the investigator from biasing the study by unintentionally selecting patients with a better prognosis for one treatment.

Unfortunately, large trials take a long time to complete, and measuring the effects on survival aren't finished until five years after the last patient is enrolled. Intermediate results from these large trials are reported as the trial progresses, but this is a lengthy process. This can be frustrating, even unfair, to someone who has to make critical decisions now.

Bottom line. You need to understand that there are different levels of certainty about experimental treatments. There are many small trials that report interesting information, some of which will hold up in further testing; some of which won't. Then there are the follow up studies, where the initial promising results are tested in multi-center trials to see whether they continue to look promising. Finally, there are the very large, multi-center, randomized trials that provide high quality answers to the issues raised in the smaller trials.

You and your treatment team need to examine the risks you face with your particular disease and make the best judgment as to whether to rely on a proven treatment or to gamble that some promising new treatment is worth staking your life on.

STATISTICAL ANALYSIS: DID IT WORK?

We would like to say "this caused that cancer." In the classic use of the word, to say that some exposure "causes" a disease implies that nearly 100% of the exposed individuals come down with it. This is an easy concept to understand, and we can predict individual outcomes using this logical framework.

Unfortunately cancer is not that simple. Even in the best studied cases, like the correlation between lung cancer and smoking, the word "cause" is inappropriate, because fewer than half of smokers develop lung cancer.

The tool for studying correlations between certain exposures and a given result is statistics.

For example, statistical arguments point out that if you count the number of cases of lung cancer among people who smoke and the number in a group who don't, the number is higher in the group who smoke. We interpret that to mean there is a risk factor associated with smoking. That is, if you smoke there is a bigger risk you will develop lung cancer.

This is not nearly so pleasing a logical framework as we would like, because it doesn't predict individual cases. Nevertheless, you need to understand something about statistics, because statistics will come up again in evaluating treatment options.

Statistical linkages should be derived from comparing groups of large numbers of cases. If there are two cases of leukemia in your neighborhood within a year, it is tempting to look for some environmental influence that may be responsible. There may be one, of course, but it could also be coincidence. If the numbers are small, there is no way to tell which. This uncertainty can lead to heated discussions and misunderstandings as to how sure we are of the correlation.

If the number of cases is large enough to make us pretty sure that it isn't just coincidence, we are able to say there is a "statistically significant" risk factor.

The rules of statistics enable us to get some measure of confidence in the finding. Let's say we are comparing two groups of people to see what proportion have some characteristic. If 90% of the people in group A have it, and only 10% in group B, then it wouldn't take many cases for us to be pretty sure that there is a significant correlation. On the other hand, if the differences are small, say 30% in one group and 33% in the other, it would take a very large number of cases to say with certainty that this isn't just due to coincidence.

This intuitive feeling is codified by statisticians in a set of rules for determining the confidence level. In essence, these rules tell you that if, you have x number of people in two groups, you can be fairly sure that the difference is real, or you can be almost positive if you have y people. How big "x" and "y" are depends on the size of the difference.

These confidence levels are an important tool in interpreting environmental hazards, as well as treatment options. The weakest confidence level is called $p = 0.1$, which means the differences are statistically significant, but not enough to give us complete confidence in the result. If $p = 0.05$, the chances are pretty good that the correlation is valid. If $p = 0.01$ or less, the result is virtually certain.

HIGH DOSE THERAPY USING STEM CELL SUPPORT

Combination therapies made up of cytotoxic drugs often kill the stem cells in your bone marrow that supply your blood cells. This results in a temporary depletion of your neutrophils (neutropenia), and/or platelets (thrombocytopenia). Recently we have developed treatments that help manage this toxicity, called growth factors, that encourage the replenishment of these cells. Growth factors represent one of the most important breakthroughs in cancer treatment, allowing us to give higher doses and, in some cases, cure patients who would not have survived otherwise.

What is a Dose?

How much drug we give is called the dose. For most drugs, the amount we give is not critical, but cancer drugs are nearly as toxic to us as they are to the tumor, and we have to be extremely cautious about how much we give.

If you are taking aspirin, chances are you take two, whether you weigh 100 lbs or 180 lbs. The amount of drug in two aspirins is the same, but the concentration is really higher in the lighter person because doses are measured as the amount of drug per pound (or kilogram) of the patient's weight. That is why children take one or one-half a tablet.

Aspirin is very safe and is effective at both concentrations, so it doesn't matter.

For some serious prescription drugs, the difference between the amount you need to be effective and the amount that could cause side effects is narrower. For these, your doctor will adjust your prescription according to your weight.

The right dose of anti-cancer drugs is even more difficult to figure. We have learned that the best way to find the right dose for different size people is not weight, but surface area. This is because a 200 lb person who is six foot five has a different physiology than a 200 lb person who is five foot tall. One way to calculate this difference is in body surface area. Experts have put together tables, in which we can find the surface area for patients with a given height and weight. In the example above, the taller patient has a surface area of 2.24, as opposed to 1.89 square meters (M^2).

Cancer drugs are usually figured in doses of drug in mg/M^2. Your dose depends on a lot of factors, such as your overall health, and what other drugs you have taken. Often, the dose is the highest your physician thinks you can tolerate. The reason is that higher doses kill more cells. You need to get to the malignant cells in the most remote part of your body with enough drug to kill every last one of them.

Increasing the Dose

We know from large clinical trials that it is necessary to exceed a threshold dose for chemotherapy to be effective. We suspect that going even higher may increase the number of patients cured, although there is some controversy over whether that is true for breast cancer. This is a hot topic today because there are new ways of increasing the impact of chemotherapy, using supportive care to modify the side effects and enable you to tolerate more drug. Before getting into this subject we need to understand what it means to increase the dose.

One way is to give the same amount of drug, but in a shorter time frame. This is called dose intensification. For example, one schedule gives 600 mg. cyclophosphamide per M^2, to be repeated after giving you three weeks to recover. We could repeat this four times (cycles), which would give you a total of 2,400 mg/M^2 in 10 weeks. If we shortened the interval between doses to two weeks, that would intensify the dose, even though we haven't changed the total amount of Cyclophosphamide. We would describe the first as 240 mg/M^2/week, and the latter as 400 mg/M^2/week.

Another way is to increase the amount of drug at each dose. In our first example, if patients could tolerate it, we could raise the dose to 1200 mg/M^2 at each dosing. If we did this for two cycles, we would be giving the same total amount as the other group got in four cycles, but we have increased the intensity.

We could also give the same dose for six cycles, increasing the cumulative dose, but not the intensity.

These three have different impacts, and you will see that we are studying them in clinical trials to determine which is best. Different physicians favor one or the other, and we cannot resolve this controversial issue yet.

Growth Factor Support

By growth factor we mean stem cell growth factor, which is not to be confused with the growth hormone HGH, designed to make short people taller.

There are several growth factor products which mimic the natural signal molecules sent to your marrow to hasten the resupply of blood cells. Providing large doses of these shortly after chemotherapy replenishes the blood much faster. Drugs like G-CSF (Filgrastim) and GM-CSF (Sargramostim) help rebuild your white blood cell counts, which does a number of good things for you. For example, it reduces the chances of your developing a serious infection, because you have more white cells to prevent it.

For another, it controls the fever of neutropenia. Your overall feeling of well being depends on constant signaling from your immune system saying "all is well." When you have too few white cells, the deficiency in signaling triggers a number of "alarm" systems, which make you feel lousy and causes various side effects, like fever. With growth factors for support, you can tolerate doses of chemotherapy between two and four times higher than you would be able otherwise.

The hope is that higher amounts of drug will kill tumor cells that would have escaped at lower doses, and increase the number of cured patients. Trials are underway to confirm this, but we don't yet have proof that stem cell support increases the cure rate. However, there is documented proof that the use of growth factors improves treatment by reducing the frequency of infection and the the symptoms, like fever and malaise, that accompanies loss of white cells.

G-CSF and GM-CSF are administered by injection under the skin. Growth factor support begins a few days after your anti-cancer treatment. This schedule is designed to wait until the toxic drugs have washed out of your marrow, and continues with daily injections for 10 to 14 days.

G-CSF and GM-CSF are two different peptide hormones, although they are both stem cell growth factors. It is easier to see the difference with a picture than it is to explain. The following illustration shows the different pathways of blood cell maturation. In the middle is the pluripotent stem cell, which can mature to become any of the mature blood cells. Down each pathway are partially mature stem cells, which wait for signal molecules to induce them to push further down the path.

As you can see, there is a major branch which produces both the monocytes and the neutrophils. GM-CSF triggers the cell which produces both neutrophils and monocytes (the one with a ✪ next to it), while G-CSF acts on the immediate precursor to the neutrophils (✳).

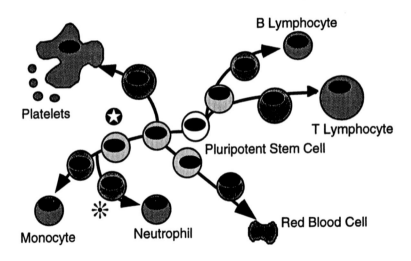

Bone Marrow Transplantation (BMT)

Allogeneic bone marrow transplant. There are two kinds of BMT, but only one is used for breast cancer.

BMT was first used to treat patients with acute leukemia. Leukemia is a malignant disease of the stem cells in the marrow. The original studies used huge dose of chemotherapy, enough to completely eliminate the cells in the patients' diseased marrow (this procedure is called ablative chemotherapy). Next they grafted new tissue, donated by close relatives, to replace the marrow. Transplant from donors whose tissue is compatible with the patients is called "allogeneic" BMT.

This procedure is used in hematologic malignancies (leukemia and lymphoma), but not for solid tumors. There are serious risks associated with ablative chemotherapy, and with rejection. The immune cells in the graft see the tissues in their new host as foreign and attempt to reject them (called graft versus host response).

For solid tumors it is often possible to remove your own marrow stem cells before starting your chemotherapy so it can be frozen and reintroduced after the therapy. This is called "autologous" BMT. Because it is your own cells that are donated, there is no risk of rejection.

With autologous BMT you can tolerate up to eight fold higher doses of chemotherapy. It is important you recognize that this is a new procedure, and it is not a cure. There are many things that can go wrong with the procedure, some of which are fatal, so it is reserved for high risk settings, where the alternatives are considered ineffective.

Techniques for autologous BMT are constantly improving, reducing both the costs and risks. More and more it is given after the first relapse. In the past, the risks were so severe it was only used in patients who had had several relapses.

If you have gone into remission after your chemotherapy, you may be given the option of being prepared for BMT. The best time to harvest your marrow is during remission, to lessen the chances your marrow contains cancer cells as well.

1   *Preparation.* You and your treatment team need to know some things before you start. You will be given several tests before you enter treatment.

   Overall health: It is important to know whether you are likely to be more sensitive to the treatment because of some underlying health problem. You will be tested to determine the condition of your heart, marrow, endocrine system, liver and kidneys as well as damage caused by previous treatments to your lungs.

   Since breast cancer often spreads to the bones, it is important to know whether there are tumors growing in your marrow before undergoing this procedure, and that will be checked thoroughly, as will other sites where the tumor might have spread.

   After high dose chemotherapy, for a period of time your immune system will completely cease to function. If you are infected with a virus, like cytomegalovirus, herpes or hepatitis, which ordinarily are kept at bay by the constant fighting of your immune system, you are likely to experience an outbreak and should receive anti-viral medication during your treatment.

   You will need to have catheters inserted in your veins to provide instant access for withdrawing blood and administering fluids and various drugs.

2   *Taking the graft.* You will be given a general anesthetic. The marrow will be removed from your hip bone by drilling a hole to provide access and flushing the marrow with a sterile saline solution. The cells will be frozen to very cold (-196° Celsius) temperatures for storage after adding an agent that preserves them through the freezing process.

3   The chemotherapy treatment is known as the conditioning regimen. For breast
     cancer this consists of combinations of one or more anti-cancer drugs at very
     high doses, and may include total body radiotherapy. Combination therapy
     includes Cyclophosphamide, Melphalan, Etoposide, Cisplatin, Thiotepa,
     Doxorubicin, Mitoxantrone and Carmustine.

        At extreme doses, the side effects of these drugs may differ from those
     experienced at "regular" doses, or be more severe. Some of these effects can be
     modified with drugs that manage side effects.

        High dose chemotherapy usually requires platelet transfusions. Currently we
     have no platelet growth factor to speed up their replenishment.

        Cyclophosphamide and Ifosfamide can cause serious side effects to the
     bladder, but that can be prevented if Mesna is administered with them.

        Skin toxicities are common. These include reddening (like sunburn),
     followed by the skin sloughing off. They also include deformed or discolored
     nail formation.

        Mucositis is also very common in high dose chemotherapy.

4   12 hours or more after the conditioning regimen your marrow cells will be
     introduced back into your body where they will recolonize the marrow and
     replenish your stem cells and circulating blood cells. How fast this happens
     depends on a number of variables, including how healthy your marrow was to
     start with, your overall health, etc. It can take as long as several months to fully
     recover.

        Among the cells in the transplant are relatively mature precursor cells. These
     are the first to develop to the point they enter your blood. On the other extreme
     are the early stem cells, which need to go through several cycles of cell
     proliferation and maturation before they produce blood cells.

        It is common to speed up the recovery process using either G-CSF or GM-
     CSF to stimulate production of new white blood cells. These are administered as
     described above.

        Another technique for speeding up the replenishment of the marrow is using
     peripheral blood progenitor cells. PBPC can be used instead of marrow cells for
     the original graft, or they can be used to supplement a marrow graft. Either way,
     the process is essentially the same as described below.

Peripheral Blood Progenitor Cells

    BMT requires special equipment and highly trained personnel, and is expensive. An
alternative procedure that has certain advantages is to collect stem cells directly from
blood withdrawn from your vein. These peripheral blood stem cells can then be
separated from other blood cells and stored so they can be grafted to your marrow after
therapy. This technique is called peripheral blood progenitor cell support (PBPC).

Peripheral blood doesn't normally contain many stem cells, but there are techniques that increase the number of circulating stem cells 100 fold. The original technique used drugs that are toxic to the bone marrow to stimulate some immature stem cells to migrate into the blood. More recently, stem cell growth factors such as G-CSF or GM-CSF are used to increase the yield of stem cells that are harvested from peripheral blood.

The procedure involves inserting a catheter into a large vein near the collar bone, so a sufficient amount of blood can be removed. The white cells are purified by a technique called leukapheresis, and you are given back your red blood cells. The purified white cells contain sufficient stem cells to repopulate the bone marrow when transfused back after the conditioning regimen. They may be further purified to eliminate any potential tumor cells accidentally picked up (called purging).

The advantages of PBPC are that the technique for gathering them is less invasive, and the recovery of the marrow is quicker than using BMT. On the other hand, the success in mobilizing PBPC varies from patient to patient. It may be necessary to collect cells from multiple cycles of harvesting to acquire sufficient numbers for the graft. BMT has been available longer, so most physicians have more confidence in it.

EXPERIMENTAL TREATMENTS FOR BREAST CANCER

This chapter will make more sense if you have read the section on Clinical Trials and Statistics first. To repeat, clinical trial data are derived from statistical arguments, and include all types of patients. No one can answer whether an individual falls into the ninety nine in one hundred category or the one in one hundred.

The process of learning how to improve treatment of cancer is a slow one. Many small trials are designed to test new drugs or ways of using them. Frequently the initial results look promising but aren't as good when tested more extensively. Large, randomized clinical trials, using many hospitals, are the gold standard for evaluating new treatments, but they take many years to complete.

The following is a report on some of the many experimental trials that are going on today. It is not an exhaustive list, but provides an idea of the alternatives that are being tested. Hopefully, it will help you understand how the clinical evaluation process works so you can read about what is the best course for you to take for your situation.

Treatment Options for Advanced Disease

1. What is the effect of estrogen on tumor growth?

A long term study followed the fate of women who had stage IV disease[9]. In advanced disease, patients whose tumor cells were estrogen receptor positive were treated in one of two groups. Some had their ovaries removed (to shut off estrogen production) and then given chemotherapy, while the other group were simply treated with chemotherapy. Removal of the ovaries made no difference to survival. In other words, the presence or absence of estrogen was not significant. This study was done in patients with stage IV disease, and we don't know for certain how it relates to early disease.

In this same study, women whose cells did not have estrogen receptors were all treated with chemotherapy. The significant finding in this study was that ER negative women had a poorer prognosis than ER positive women.

2. Does it do any good to treat advanced disease?

We know that treating Stage 0, I and II disease produces a high number of cures, but it is not obvious whether chemotherapy improves survival in the more advanced stages of disease. The current feeling is that at the least, chemotherapy improves the quality of life in these patients, and there is growing evidence that new techniques, such as <u>bone marrow transplant</u>, are increasing the number of responses. When we have had longer to study these women who responded, we may see an increase in survival.

3. How do you evaluate the effectiveness of adjuvant chemotherapy?

These authors[10] looked at historical data from many clinical trials in premenopausal women whose cancer had spread to their lymph nodes. They found that adjuvant chemotherapy reduces the odds of recurrence by 36% and reduces death by 25%. That is, the number of deaths is 25% less in a group of patients who were treated with chemotherapy than in a group who were not treated.

In ten years, these figures mean a 12% difference in disease free survival between the treated and untreated groups, and a 10% difference in overall survival[11]. A 10% difference may not seem dramatic at first, but it means that thousands of women survived because of chemotherapy.

In post-menopausal women, the differences are slightly lower. For example the ten year overall survival difference between groups who were treated and those who weren't is 7%. Of course post-menopausal women are older, so their ten year life expectancy is lower, whether or not they have cancer.

If you look at nodal status, classifying patients as node negative (0) or node positive (+), there is a 70% improvement in ten year overall survival in patients who are node positive and underwent chemotherapy. It is worth mentioning that this study included all types of chemotherapy, including combinations that are not as effective as those we use today.

The bottom line is that chemotherapy saves lives.

4. How should Tamoxifen be used?

A mathematical analysis was done to see whether tamoxifen improves the chances of overall survival. This study showed that node + women treated with Tamoxifen will benefit more than node 0 women. This enigma is one of those common sense traps we get into with statistics. It doesn't mean that node 0 women shouldn't use Tamoxifen. The reason it appears to work better in node + women is because their risk is greater.

Tamoxifen is more effective against tumors that are receptor positive, although there is a survival benefit in receptor negative tumors, too. (Some argue this is impossible. They insist that the receptor negative women who responded were actually receptor positive, but the test used to classify their receptor status was wrong.)

These data include early trials where Tamoxifen was used for only 1 year, which may not have been optimal. It is not clear at this point when women should discontinue Tamoxifen, but the trend is to treat at least two years. Whether treatment for longer improves the risk of survival is not yet known.

Tamoxifen works better in elderly patients than it does in younger patients[12]. Again, this doesn't really mean better. It means older women have a higher risk, and benefited more than younger women. What it says is that women over 65 obtain substantial benefit from Tamoxifen.

There is reason to be concerned that Tamoxifen use can lead to other health problems. You have to decide what the chances of these other health problems are, for you, versus the chances of keeping your cancer from returning.

5. Do women who have undergone treatment feel that it was worth it?

In this study, women who had undergone chemotherapy were polled to find out what risk conditions would convince them to undergo it again. Their answer (not surprising) depended on how much benefit they could expect. The greater the improvement in ten year survival, the more likely they would undergo treatment. This study established realistic boundary conditions from a population that is in the best position to know. The authors also found that older women required more palpable benefits than younger women.

6. Does giving more chemotherapy improve survival?

This is one of the important controversies in cancer treatment today. To achieve full survival benefits, it is important to deliver the full dose of chemotherapy. The CALGB 8541 trial[13] was designed to answer this question, although we have made so much progress since this trial was designed, the results may not pertain to today's treatments.

In this study they looked at three doses of FAC every four weeks for 4 cycles. The three treatment groups were given doses of either (600/60/600) vs. (400/40/400) vs.

(300/30/300). Disease free survival as well as overall survival are reduced in the low dose arm. However, the differences between the two higher doses are not significant.

This study shows that reducing the dose (because patients have trouble tolerating the full schedule) should be avoided if at all possible. It does not prove that increasing the dose beyond this threshold is better. It is worth noting that this study was set up before the use of growth factor support, so it doesn't address the question of what happens when you increase the dose of FAC even higher.

A similar trial is ongoing[14] from the NSABP. This trial does not include the use of stem cell support to boost the dose intensity, either.

7. Is there a way of predicting whether chemotherapy will be beneficial?

There are several genetic markers that could someday be used to help predict who will benefit from therapy, or even which therapy will work best. *HER-2/neu* is one example of these. Several small scale studies have shown that patients whose tumor cells contain multiple copies of the oncogene HER-2/neu[15] do not respond well to chemotherapy[16]. However, most oncologists wouldn't withhold chemotherapy until more data appear or a better alternative is presented.

These tests are new, and many physicians have questions about the reproducibility, standardization, availability and cost of these tests. Evaluating diagnostic procedures in randomized studies would help convince physicians of their value. However, it is going to be difficult to initiate trials because it is too early to commit to the 10 years that will be required to test a marker when new discoveries may make it obsolete next year.

8. It is generally accepted that combinations of different drugs are more effective than single agents. Are some combinations more effective than others?

The impression from large scale trials seems to indicate that combinations that include one of the anthracycline family of drugs are better than those that do not. However, one randomized study in 500 patients compared CMF with CAF[17], and found no significant difference in survival after five years. A similar international study in 760 patients compared CMF with FEC[18], again showing no significant difference.

More recent studies done in Canada[19] and Italy[20] showed better results for groups treated with a combination containing one of the anthracyclines. Additional studies may resolve this discrepancy. As of today, these studies have convinced many (but not all) oncologists there is a better cure rate for combinations with anthracyclines.

9. Is Neoadjuvant therapy better than the standard sequence?

Neoadjuvant therapy means treating with chemotherapy prior to surgery or radiotherapy to reduce the tumor size and kill cells in metastases before excision. Sometimes oncologists describe it as "downsizing" the tumor. One of the theories behind neoadjuvant therapy is that we have a better chance of eliminating metastases if the chemotherapy is given before the trauma of surgery or radiotherapy.

This is a relatively new approach, and has shown promising results in other types of cancer, such as Non-Small Cell Lung Cancer. It is being tested by the NSABP in an ongoing trial[21], but it is too early yet to interpret the results. A French group is using neoadjuvant therapy in combination with other drugs to treat large local tumors[22]. It is well worth following the results of these trials as more patients enroll in the studies.

10. Once treatment is completed, do you improve overall survival by intensive scheduling of follow up visits and testing patients frequently?

This study showed that a group of patients who were tested and examined frequently for relapses[23] had no survival benefit over a group left alone. This counter-intuitive finding has important consequences both for controlling health care costs and patients' peace of mind.

Experimental trials: New Drugs

There are a number of new agents that are available for testing. Of these, the taxanes are considered to have the most potential. Navelbine is well tolerated, so it may develop a rôle, perhaps in combination with 5-FU. Topotecan is severely myelosuppressive, and as such difficult to combine with other drugs.

1. Mitoxantrone is a relatively new agent that is tolerated better than most anthracyclines[24]. This study shows that as a single agent it is active, but not better than CMFP.

Mitoxantrone has been approved in Canada for eight years, and has become part of some standard therapies. In the US it is currently being evaluated in combination with other drugs[25].

2. Taxol is a very promising new agent, but it causes severe neutropenia. Almost all new agents are being tested with growth factors to increase the dose[26] and maximize the potential benefit. Combination studies to find the best ways of using Taxol are underway[27],[28].

We know Taxol and Taxotere are active as single agents, and the next step is to find out how to use them with other drugs. The next generation of studies with Taxotere should be combined with growth factor support.

It is still too early to think of the taxanes for front-line therapy. There is a lot of toxicity, especially with the higher doses.

3. Goserelin is an LHRH agonist initially approved for prostate cancer and then expanded to include treatment of endometriosis. It is now being tested to see whether it can be used like Tamoxifen for hormonal control of disease[29].

4. Aredia is a Bisphosphonate used to control a side effect of advanced disease, hypercalcemia. Bisphosphonate imitates the inorganic component of bones, and controls

bone absorption. There is a study in patients whose disease has spread to the bone to see whether Aredia has any effect on controlling their disease[30]. This study showed Bisphosphonate was well tolerated and appeared to slow disease progression.

5.   Lonidamine is an agent designed to block the multi drug resistance activity in cells that have become resistant to anti-cancer drugs. It improves anthracycline cytotoxicity by increasing the intracellular concentration of drug[31] in resistant cells. This study will show whether it is as effective in people as it was in the laboratory.

6.   Navelbine is another new agent that was recently approved by the FDA. It does not seem to be as active as the taxanes, although that is a consensus impression, and more studies may prove otherwise. As an oral drug[32] it is easier for older people to take and is less toxic. It is a useful agent in anthracycline resistant settings.

In combination with 5-FU patients had serious mucositis, with no obvious benefit compared with other regimens[33].

7.   Toremifene is a new drug designed to have less side effects and work as well as Tamoxifen[34].

8.   Liposomes. Anthracyclines, such as Doxorubicin, Epirubicin, Idarubicin and Mitoxantrone, are active against breast cancer, and are often used as one of the main ingredients in a combination "cocktail" of drugs. All anthracyclines can cause irreversible damage to the heart muscle if used too much. This is a serious problem, and limits how high the dose can be increased. One idea for overcoming this problem is to put the anthracycline inside a liposome so it doesn't get at the heart muscle. Preliminary results indicate this idea may work in practice[35], although the number of patients studied is still small.

Dose Intensification Studies

We are searching for an effective way to treat women with advanced disease. We believe the best hope is to combine several drugs with radiation and/or surgery and use them as aggressively as possible. Stem cell support allows you to receive higher doses of cytotoxic agents, but does that increase your chances of surviving this disease?

An Italian group has developed a three tiered approach to treating their patients who have more than 10 lymph nodes involved[36]. They have seen encouraging results for overall survival, so far, and are about to begin a randomized trial.

Most experimental studies are done with women who have advanced disease, have relapsed, and been treated at least once, often several times. People who have failed other treatments are the most difficult to cure, and it is hard to draw conclusions about how these therapies would work in previously untreated advanced disease.

Some opinion leaders believe that dose intensification is leading to increased numbers of cured patients, and are enthusiastic that the rates will be remarkable as this treatment option is used early in the course of treatment.

However, others have concluded that neither single agent, high dose chemotherapy with alkylating agents nor combinations of agents offer patients with breast cancer significant long term survival benefit, even when given at doses that are only possible with autologous BMT[37].

This paper reviews the data from several small trials in patients with node negative Stage IV disease where high dose consolidation was used. Some of these trials used doses that required BMT or PBPC, (ablative), and some that used only growth factors (subablative). Efficacy was measured in conversion from partial to complete response, disease free survival, and overall survival.

Various drug combinations and target groups for trials were compared. Most studies increased the proportion of patients who are free of disease after two years from 17 to 26%. This looks good compared to the expected rate of 10%, although there were a number of treatment related deaths. If these results continue as more patients receive this treatment, it will change the overall statistics.

The emerging trend is to initiate with standard dose chemotherapy, and move those who respond to high dose consolidation. The results suggest some of these patients achieve a durable response[38].

Managing the effect on the bone marrow toxicity with G-CSF allows us to raise the dose above what patients normally could tolerate. Early results in one study[39] appear very promising. It also allows us to administer the dose with shorter recovery periods between doses[40]. This study showed that interval reduction lead to a dose intensity increase of 2 to 1.

It is worth pointing out in these dose intensive therapies for metastatic diseases thrombocytopenia is severe. For example in one study, every patient needed platelet transfusions. This underlines the need for an additional stem cell factor to replenish platelets.

In practice, dose escalation with stem cell support is being adopted before the randomized clinical trial data are available to evaluate the efficacy and safety of the procedures[41]. It will be very important to test this in randomized clinical trials, since this could be the treatment of choice within 5 years.

In the US, fewer than 10% of the women with Stage I or II disease who are receiving autologous stem cell support are participating in randomized clinical trials, and fewer than 5% of patients with metastatic disease are in clinical trials. Without randomized clinical trials, we cannot get definitive answers to the crucial questions we have about treatment options.

What tests help predict what is going to happen?

The subset of people who fare best with Stage II breast cancer are those with the least node involvement. Over 85% of patients with more than 4 nodes involved will relapse[42]. Other prognostic factors are: poorly differentiated tumors, distorted chromosomes, a high proportion of cells in S phase, and an excessive copy number of HER-2/neu genes.

Stage III is locally advanced with no evidence of metastasis. Any size tumor where the nodal status is 2 or 3 is now considered unresectable. These are patients who have a poor prognosis and should be entered in experimental trials.

Inflammatory breast cancer is a less common disease, where the breast is enlarged, indurated and has invaded subdermal lymphatics. There is no standard therapy. We don't know how to treat these patients with a high probability of success. One institute reports a reasonable success rate with a combined therapy approach[43]. We don't know yet whether this rate will be seen in other hospitals.

What about the cost of treatment?

High dose chemotherapy with autologous stem cell support in breast cancer represents 35% of all bone marrow transplants done in the US[44]. The cost is $50,000 to $150,000 per patient, with 20,000 potential patients.

These authors estimate high dose chemotherapy adds 9.6 months to the life of the average woman, at a cost of $100,000/life year. This compares with $50,000/life year for kidney dialysis. While pricing models are being studied, there is no answer to what costs are acceptable. Extensive trials are underway to give firm numbers to the analysis.

5

MANAGING SIDE EFFECTS

Cancer treatment is nearly as debilitating as the disease itself. Some of the side effects of radiotherapy or chemotherapy can hurt you terribly. As you've learned, this is because cancer cells are nearly indistinguishable from healthy ones, so the treatment is going to disrupt some healthy cells as a side effect.

The following sections describe how the effects on your cells translate into the side effects you feel. Some of these are severe, even lethal, and others are emotionally disturbing, even though they may not be life threatening.

It is important you understand the struggle that is going on between your body and the deranged cells that made the tumor. Understanding can help you cope, and regain control over your body. Focus inward and try to sense the healing process. This is a spiritual dimension, and different people approach it from each their unique perspective. Whatever way works for you, take control.

This is a battle for your life. When you are able to focus on your health, you will put the side effects in perspective. Preparation will make side effects less severe, and help you regain control of your body during the treatment. Therapy helps fight the disease, but above all, you need to nurture your body's response. In the process you will gain confidence and restore order over the depredations of this chaos inside you.

TAKE CONTROL

We tend to focus on the tumor itself as the key to cancer, it is important to recognize that there are other factors as well. Cancer cells cannot grow without support from other, healthy cells. Somehow, these cells have to be duped by the cancer into helping.

Blood vessels have to develop to increase the flow of nourishment to a tumor and dispose of the waste products produced during growth. The surrounding tissue, called the stroma, provides a supportive environment for the tumor to grow. Stromal cells rearrange the structure of the tissue to allow the tumor to grow, and they nourish the tumor by bathing it in a supportive communication network. Rejection by immune system also has to be subverted to prevent the killer cells from infiltrating and destroying the tumor.

All these interconnected systems interact to help the tumor grow despite the threat to your health. The point is, you have a certain amount of control over them.

The ultimate expression of the dynamics of the interaction of the myriad systems operating in your body is your mood. Normally thousands of little events go on without you knowing, but when things are slipping out of control, your body sends an alarm. That alarm consists of a signal that interrupts your mood, to influence your behavior in a way that will be best for your health.

For example, when your immune system is fighting an infection, you feel miserable. If it is severe you develop a fever, because your white cells give off a signal that acts directly on the brain to cause fever. You ache all over because your immune system gives off another, different signal that acts on your muscles. These signals have the effects of causing you to go off somewhere safe and rest for a few days, to help your immune system fight the infection.

The immune system is only one of the networks that can influence your mind. Your mood is affected by many other systems that normally operate without your being aware, but which can affect your mood when the situation calls for it.

As your body lets you know about your wellness by affecting your mood, you have the ability to reverse this process, and influence your health through your mind. You need to alter these systems and redirect them into a mode of action that will help heal you.

How you accomplish this depends on your personal background. We are not accustomed to thinking about health as something we can manipulate, but there is ample evidence that it's possible. In the East, cults of mysticism and meditation, such as yoga, have long been able to influence the body through the mind. Western traditions of healing through faith demonstrate similar feats by different means.

In other words, there are different paths to the same end. You need to find a path that fits your beliefs and values to achieve wellness. Whether that is through a consummate faith in a supreme being acting upon your body, a transcendence through meditation, a ritual of diet, or a faith in science is immaterial. Each works for certain people, depending on their background.

What you are seeking begins with confidence that you can redirect the struggle going on inside you. You need to exercise your willpower to establish a mood that emanates a dominant sense of well-being and power over the systems that guide you with subliminal messages. As these networks affect your mood, so can you affect them by imposing a sense of wellness and control over them.

Reasserting control over your body is not a substitute for the best tools of medicine, but it does supplement your therapy and potentiate it. Learning about your disease, what's going on inside you and how therapy is going to disrupt your body may help. If you are prepared for what is coming, you will handle it better, maintain a dominant mood of being in control, and help your body fight cancer.

Try to spend at least thirty minutes each day tuning in to your body. Whether you elect meditation or prayer, learn to feel the subtle signals going on inside you. Find a quiet time, away from distraction, and compose yourself. Calm your emotions, and strive to feel inside yourself. As you learn to tune in to your body, begin to assert control. You need to emanate a sense of peace and bliss, and send a message back through these communication channels that you are well, that you are in control, and that what is wrong needs to be righted.

Your therapy may involve treatment with drugs and radiation. You should learn about the side effects you will experience and prepare as best you can for the assaults on your body. This is a desperate struggle, and you will feel its effects. Steel yourself, and ride the storm so you can establish control again as soon as possible. The less time you spend succumbing to these side effects, the better you will be able to fight your disease.

DIET

The influence of diet on cancer is a controversial subject. There a number of books by cancer survivors or nutritionists that make extravagant claims about the value of their product. Many oncologists tend to be skeptical that these diets are effective in large groups of patients. They know that tumors sometimes disappear spontaneously, and they assume that the authors of these books are misinterpreting spontaneous remission for diet therapy.

There are no clinical studies that support diet as a therapy for cancer. Diet may help your body fight the cancer, but it is not a substitute for standard therapy. The best advice is to follow the medical professionals.

However, diet can be one of the weapons you use to draw up the resources of your body. First of all you should eat enough to keep you healthy. This can be difficult, since some treatments make you nauseous. Nevertheless, you have to keep your weight up and provide all the nutrients your body needs, otherwise your immune system will be weakened.

You should eat foods that are strong stimulants for your immune system and foods that contain compounds that effect your DNA repair systems. Your diet should include foods that contain the germinal material, because seeds are rich in enzymes, bioflavonoids, vitamins and cofactors that affect DNA. This includes nuts, seeds, beans, and fruits that contain seeds. Plant roots are also rich in growth factors, so include sprouts, carrots, potato skins and wheat germ.

Many seeds are designed to pass intact through an animal's digestive system as part of their natural history. To obtain the full benefit of the nutrients in these seeds, you must open them, either mechanically, or by roasting or frying in a hot skillet. One less tasty solution to this problem is to obtain pulverized seed products.

Plants also contain a rich armament of chemicals that prevent decay. While its effects are similar to our immune system, it is completely different. Plants protect themselves with myriad antibiotics that repel or injure invading fungi and bacteria. Some of these compounds are stimulants of our own immune system. They are found in vegetables like broccoli, cauliflower, root vegetables and unpolished rice.

Mucositis/Stomatitis

The sheath lining the digestive tract, called the mucosa, is very sensitive to radiation and some drugs. Inflammation of the mucosa is called mucositis, which can become ulcerated and the stomach or intestines can be perforated. The mucosa also includes the lining of mouth; sometimes inflammation of the mucosa of the mouth is called stomatitis. In most cases, the painful damage to the gums and oral tissues is the most noticeable, although the entire mucosa may be affected.

Stomatitis usually lasts for a short time, but can be extremely painful. You should prepare ahead of time if you are going to receive radiation therapy whose port includes the oral cavity or if your chemotherapy includes drugs that are likely to cause it.

You need to keep your mouth clean and moist. Your mouth is full of bacteria which can cause serious problems if they get into your blood while your white cells are depleted. Fungi from your mouth are another source of blood infections. Usually a dentist will examine you prior to your treatment to make sure the flora growing in your mouth are under control and won't get into your blood through ulcers of the skin.

You should be particularly careful to keep your teeth and gums free of plaque during your treatment. Frequent brushing and flossing are important. If your gums are too sensitive for brushing, try toothpastes that contain baking soda, or hydrogen peroxide. You may wish to use Q-tips, a Water-Pik or Toothettes instead of a brush.

Most mouthwashes have a lot of alcohol in them, which is the last thing you need when your mouth is dry. There are commercial products designed to keep your mouth moist, or you can prepare your own. Slightly salty water, or baking soda dissolved in water work well. You may want to include some topical analgesic, like lidocaine, xylocaine or benzocaine.

Candies that induce salivation are another good idea. Some hospitals prepare popsicles with Nystatin frozen in water as a way to control pain and provide a topical antibiotic. There are also salves prepared specifically for covering mouth sores.

You can speed up the recovery of the oral mucosa with a highly nutritious diet, including lots of proteins (eggs, milk, and cheese or meat that has been prepared in a blender). Milk shakes, macaroni and cheese are examples of foods that are soothing and nutritious. Avoid alcohol, tobacco or foods that are spicy or acidic, like fruits.

Fatigue

Cancer and cancer treatments can cause a debilitating fatigue that may last for months after therapy. Many patients find fatigue the most serious side effect of their disease, although it doesn't appear threatening to some physicians. The cause may be depression, energy depletion in the central nervous system or an interruption of one of the many as yet undiscovered signal systems that control how we feel about ourselves.

The effects of fatigue tend to snowball, as people feel more lethargic, which puts the burden of care on those around them, who also become fatigued and depressed. Try to be aware of the strain on those around you and try to cope with your fatigue as a side effect of your disease that is treatable, and don't let it become your normal behavior.

Nutrition can be part of the problem. Cancer cells are competing for nutrients, treatment depletes your cells which need to regrow quickly, and this all taxes your energy reserves.

Sometimes fatigue is due to an inability to sleep which may be remedied with a change in habits. Exercising may also help.

APPETITE

Like fatigue, loss of appetite and the sometimes dramatic weight loss that accompanies cancer and its treatment is probably due to interruption of some of the signal systems that operate constantly to affect how we feel about ourselves. We know that Tumor Necrosis Factor (TNF), a cytokine emitted by macrophages, can cause severe weight loss (cachexia) in laboratory animals. We suspect that TNF given off by our immune system's fight against the cancer may operate on our fat storage centers.

Since nutrition contributes to many of the side effects, it is important to get back control of your appetite. Medication that help include Prednisone® Megace® or Marinol®.

EMESIS (NAUSEA)

Nausea and/or vomiting are a common side effect of many anti-cancer drugs. In some patients vomiting is so severe it prevents them from continuing their treatments.

Our understanding of the physiology behind nausea has grown in recent years, as researchers work to develop drugs to overcome the reaction. The reflex protects us from becoming sick when we eat noxious foods. It is designed to purge the stomach when we happen to eat a mushroom or plant that might kill us.

The sequence starts when conditions stimulate a cell in the intestines to send a signal molecule that provokes the nervous system and initiates the response. The reaction involves a complex series of reactions, including perspiration, loss of equilibrium, and salivation. It culminates in the sequential contractions of the stomach muscle, opening the pyloric valve and so on. This series of events involve systems throughout our body, which coordinate as though the brain plays a preprogrammed cassette, which is exactly the case.

The sequence of reactions is controlled from a region in the brain called the vomiting center. Some anti-cancer drugs work directly on this center, but most operate on one or more of the nerves that make up the signal network which triggers the reaction center in the brain.

Our conscious mind has some control over emesis, but it is important you understand it is a natural response, provoked by the drug stimulating one of the cells that transmit the chain of signals in the nervous system. Responses differ in individuals and at different doses. The drugs that often cause severe vomiting are given in the following table. Those in the bottom section induce emesis about half the time. The table also gives you a rough idea when it will start and how long it is likely to last.

You can prepare ahead of time for treatment. If you are tense or upset, it will contribute to the severity of the reaction. As best you can, calm yourself before hand. Counseling is helpful, and your care givers may suggest relaxation exercises such as meditation, yoga, hypnosis or alternatives that condition you for a smoother therapy.

You should expect some nausea, and eat and drink enough far ahead of time so you won't suffer from fluid or weight loss. Avoid foods that are even mildly upsetting during the time of your therapy.

Emetic Drugs

Drug	Onset (hours)	Duration (hours)
Cisplatin	4	24 - 240
Dacarbazine	2	1 - 12
Mechlorethamine	2	8 - 36
Carmustine or Lomustine	3	4 - 24
Cyclophosphamide	8	4 - 10
Cytarabine	9	3 - 5
Dactinomycin	4	12 - 24
Methotrexate	4	3 - 24
5-Fluorouracil	5	3 - 24
Mitomycin C	1	48 - 72
Carboplatin	6	18 - 24
Doxorubicin or Epirubicin	5	6
Bleomycin	5	12
Etoposide	5	12
Ifosfamide	1	12
Melphalan	9	12
Mercaptopurine	6	8
Teniposide	5	6
Thiotepa	9	12
Vincristine or Vinblastine	6	24

Many patients become sensitized to throwing up after the first dose. When this happens, any one of a hundred little details that remind them of their treatment can cause them to get sick. Things associated with treatment, like the color of the room, or smells, or even faces can stimulate the reaction.

If you are receiving treatment at home, avoid cooking odors by having your food prepared elsewhere. Try to put yourself in surroundings that you won't find yourself in again once the treatment is over so you won't be reminded of the therapy. Don't eat your favorite foods until after your therapy is complete, because you may end up associating them with the treatment.

Medicines to Control Emesis

One effective way of controlling nausea is to make you a little woozy with drugs like Lorazepam or Diazepam. We have learned that patients who don't remember everything about their treatment are less likely to trigger vomiting through associations. They will also be less likely to stop therapy because of intolerance to the emetic side effects.

Metaclopromide is an anti-emetic drug that is often combined with Lorazepam. It has its own side effects, like making you feel dizzy or restless.

Glucocorticoids, like dexamethasone, also help control emesis, especially when combined with other agents.

Some tranquilizers, like Haloperidol and Droperidol, are also effective at controlling emesis in some patients. Another class of tranquilizers that have been tested as effective anti-emetics includes prochlorperazine and thiethylperazine. At higher doses, however, all these cause side effects which limit their use.

Ondansetron (brand name Zofran®) is an effective anti-emetic compound, but is very expensive and must be administered by intravenous injection. In settings where none of the others work, Ondansetron has helped many patients control their emesis. It is designed to prevent the signal molecule sent from the small intestine from binding to its receptor and stimulating the brain to cause the vomiting reflex.

Marijuana derivatives, like Marinol, are sometimes used. They cause a euphoric sensation that some find pleasant, and for these patients the drugs are useful. However, most patients dislike the euphoric sensation, and prefer other drugs.

Antihistamines are less potent than other anti-emetics. Since they cause few side effects, antihistamines like Diphenhydramine can be added to combinations to make them more effective.

CONSTIPATION

Certain drugs used in chemotherapy and some pain medications affect the movement of your intestines which causes constipation. It is important to keep ahead of this reaction to prevent impaction. Impaction is a very hard, large stool that is difficult to pass, and causes real distress you don't want to deal with. An impaction gets worse the longer it persists because your intestines are constantly extracting water from the stool, making it harder and harder.

This is one side effect that can be prevented. There are lots of laxatives and stool softeners that will keep constipation under control. Your care givers will help you with appropriate medicines; the important thing is to be sure to keep ahead of this side effect, lest you develop a serious problem.

NEPHROTOXICITY

Your kidneys are a major organ in the waste removal system that keeps you healthy. Most people know that the kidneys remove certain waste products from the blood which are transferred to the bladder for elimination as urine. A critical role for the kidneys is eliminating excess nitrogen, which is left over after we transform food into the energy that keeps us alive. Nitrogen is transformed into a chemical called urea for easy disposal. Without the constant cleansing of nitrogen from the blood we would be dead in a few hours, so it is vitally important to monitor kidney function and prevent renal failure.

Blood consists of cells, mostly red blood cells, suspended in a fluid called serum (also known as plasma). As blood passes through the special vessels in the kidneys, some serum is removed on its way through the capillaries. In the average person the kidneys remove over 4 gallons of liquid a day. Almost all of this fluid is quickly put back in, and the portion that doesn't flows into the bladder as urine.

During this, the serum is cleansed. The liquid and much of the substances dissolved in it, are filtered as it passes through special cells, which return it back to the blood. During this, most harmful byproducts go out with the urine for excretion.

Drugs like Cisplatin, or Pentostatin, become toxic inside the cells which are performing this filtration. When they do, it can be catastrophic, even fatal. We have learned that increasing the rate of flow by overloading the body with fluids reduces the time of exposure to the drug in these cells and lessens the nephrotoxicity.

You may be given a lot of water to drink and/or intravenous fluids to increase the amount of urine from about a pint a day to several quarts.

Drugs like Ifosfamide or Cyclophosphamide can produce a substance called acrolein that collects in the bladder. Acrolein is toxic and may cause bladder cancer. Fortunately, the drug Mesna neutralizes acrolein. Mesna is often given along with chemotherapy using these drugs for this reason.

Some of the tests done on your blood measure chemicals that tell us that your kidneys are not functioning properly long before you have any symptoms. If you notice blood in your urine you should notify your physician.

NEUTROPENIA

If you look at a drop of blood in the microscope, you will see it contains lots of red blood cells, platelets, and a few white cells. When stained with dyes designed to enhance the visibility of tissues in the microscope, you will see these white cells are not all the same.

The most common cell type are called either neutrophils (just to confuse the issue they also go by another name of polymorphonuclear cells). Neutrophils are the patrol cars of the blood; the first defense against foreign invaders. They need to be replenished often because they only live for one or two days. As they circulate in the blood, they are primed to respond to trouble. Either signals from other cells or contact with abnormal conditions can trigger them to respond.

They contain hundreds of disease fighting tool kits which they can use, depending on the situation. We are only beginning to understand the repertoire of tricks neutrophils use to fight off invaders, but we know they can kill other cells with some of the substances they give off. They also send alarms to other cells to summon help to control the situation. They may call up more neutrophils, or other cells, or they may change the blood flow locally by signaling the cells lining the blood vessels to open up and let fluid flow into the tissue.

Both chemotherapy drugs and radiotherapy can kill the stem cells in the marrow that replenish neutrophils. When the laboratory finds your white counts have fallen below 1,500 cells per cubic millimeter you are neutropenic. The severity of your neutropenia depends on how low the cell counts go (see toxicity table at the end of this book).

Without neutrophils you are much more likely to develop infections than you would normally. This vulnerability to bacterial or fungal infection is a serious problem and kills many patients each year. Sources of infection include bacteria or yeast in your mouth, which ordinarily are not dangerous but take advantage of the opportunity presented because your immune system is not functioning properly. You can also get infections from contact with contaminated surfaces, or breathing aerosolized germs.

There are other side effects from neutropenia that are related to the absence of this important system of cells that are involved in many signal networks which regulate your health. These include fever, and an overall feeling that you are really, really sick.

Supportive care is available to shorten the length of time you are neutropenic using stem cell support. This reduces the risk of your developing an infection, shortens the time you need to stay in the hospital and makes you feel better. It also helps you by allowing you to tolerate more of the drugs used to fight your cancer.

PAIN

Pain is not always part of cancer. Anticipating pain is often worse than the event, so it is important to understand that many cancer patients never experience pain from their disease or its treatment.

Pain can be produced directly by a tumor, as its growth impacts on nerves. Cancer that has spread to the bones, for example, often is painful. Stomach and intestinal cancer also can affect the nerves.

Pain can be caused directly by all types of therapy: surgery, radiotherapy and some of the drugs used in chemotherapy. It can also arise from pressure building up due to blockage in lymphatic flow. Mouth sores, too, can be painful until they heal.

Many types of pain can be controlled with narcotics. If you are experiencing pain, let your doctor know. It may be telling him important information about your body and its response to your disease and treatment.

A lot of patients are reserved about their pain, for a number of different reasons. You are in a war for control over your body. Don't weaken yourself by fighting pain as well as your disease.

Some are afraid they will become addicted to the narcotics. This should not be a concern. Pain has serious effects on your feeling of well being and your ability to recover. It is much more important that you control your pain, no matter how much it takes.

Pain control starts with mild drugs, and only escalates to stronger medications if it gets worse. If your pain gets to the point it needs strong drugs, like morphine, to manage it while you're getting better, don't hesitate to use them. Addiction to narcotics used for pain control is very different than it is for people trying to get "high." Don't worry about it.

Some patients are shy about pain. Don't be. It isn't a test of your ability to endure, it is a symptom of your body not working right. There is a curious psychology about pain and prescribing medications to control it. Some patients, even some doctors, feel guilty about treating pain. This guilt may come from their attitude to "secret pleasures," and is not relevant to cancer treatment. Use whatever means are necessary to control it, so you can focus on restoring your sense of well being.

One type of pain, called neuropathic pain, is caused by damage to nerves. Neuropathic pain usually does not respond to narcotics, and other types of therapy, like nerve blocks, are required.

THE LYMPHATIC SYSTEM AND EDEMA

While people are familiar with the bloodstream, not everyone is aware that there is a second circulatory system called the lymph system. Unlike the closed loop of the bloodstream, the lymphatic is an open ended network. It funnels fluid from all tissues through a network of lymph vessels that fuse into larger lymph vessels, which fuse again, eventually to collect in a reservoir that empties it into the blood.

As blood cells rush through the capillaries, some of the fluid seeps through the capillary walls and escapes the bloodstream. You've seen this serous fluid as the clear, slightly yellow liquid that comes out of healing cuts. Normally, it seeps through the tiny spaces in all tissues, collecting in open ended lymphatic vessels that vacuum up this fluid. The purpose of the lymphatic flow is to collect debris and sweep the tissues with antibodies present in the fluid. The lymphatic vessels are studded everywhere with small chambers called lymph nodes. The lymph nodes check the fluid for foreign matter and protect you from contaminants that might have gotten into your body. When there is an active infection, they enlarge, as everyone knows.

Because they are a channel through which things flow, lymph nodes are one of the paths that cells take when they break off a tumor and spread. This is why your doctor checks the lymph nodes along the path that flows from a tumor. Hopefully, any spreading will be confined to these nodes, and can be removed by surgery or killed with radiation.

Experience has taught us that often the first site into which breast cancer cells spread is the cluster of lymph nodes under your arm, the axillary nodes. From there, cells may spread to the lymph nodes around your collar bone.

The volume of fluid that flows through the lymphatic system is larger than you might expect. When a cluster of vessels is removed, the fluid upstream of the block has no place to go. As fluid backs up, the tissues swell, a condition called edema. Eventually your body will make a new pathway so this fluid can get around the block, but until it does, edema can be painful and disconcerting.

THROMBOCYTOPENIA

Platelets, or thrombocytes, are tiny cell parts in the blood whose main function is to trigger clotting. They are not cells, but pieces of a very large cell (megakaryocyte) in the bone marrow whose job is to produce bags of chemicals which pinch off then enter the bloodstream. Platelets have no DNA, and therefore cannot reproduce.

The chemicals they contain combine with proteins in the blood to form a clot when there is a leak in a blood vessel. Their surface is triggered to make them stick to the vessel wall, and they release substances that quickly produce fibers which act as molecular "rebars" to staunch the flow of blood and stimulate the repair process.

Some anti-cancer drugs kill the megakaryocytes and cut off the replacement of new platelets. When the number of platelets falls below 100,000 cells per cubic millimeter, you can have medical problems due to poor clotting and this condition is called thrombocytopenia.

The lower the counts, the less well you will form clots. This can be serious, but you can control some of the risk by avoiding situations where you might be cut or bruised.

Stem cells in the marrow will eventually replace the megakaryocytes, and the platelet counts will return to normal. How fast this happens will depend on the drug, your health, and other things.

We don't have a growth factor to stimulate replenishing the platelets. Some experimental drugs being studied in the clinic, like Interleukin-11 and PIXY-321, appear to act as platelet growth factors along with other effects they produce. They need more study before they can be approved for this purpose. There are also two candidates for platelet growth factors that are nearly ready for testing in clinical trials.

Hair loss (Alopecia) and Nail Changes

The cells that make hair and those that make your finger and toe nails are some of the most active cells in the body. For this reason, they are also very sensitive to many of the drugs used in chemotherapy. Usually the hair follicle cells don't die, but they become "sick" enough to stop making hair temporarily, and the hair often falls out as a result. Usually hair grows back, although sometimes it will have a different color.

The cells in your nail bed are also disrupted, and the result is malformed nail during the time of your chemotherapy. You will see a ridge or discoloration in your fingernails that takes months to grow out.

Hair loss can be devastating, psychologically. At best, hair loss and nail ridges are a constant reminder of something you would like to forget. Many patients find the loss of their hair more devastating than any of the life threatening events during their treatment.

Unfortunately, we do not yet have the ability to prevent either of these. Hospitals often apply "ice caps" to chill the surface and try to reduce the metabolism of the hair cells so they won't be as sensitive to the chemotherapy drugs. While this is worth trying, it doesn't work very well, and you had better prepare yourself for the chance that you will lose your hair.

It is a good idea to purchase a wig prior to undergoing treatment. These may be uncomfortable, but allow you to socialize without provoking scrutiny. Some prefer a turban as an alternative. A silk pillowcase is less abrasive, and may keep some hair from coming out during sleep.

Reconstructive Surgery

Surgical removal of a breast often is deeply traumatic. Surgeons have developed amazing techniques for reconstructing the breast, including the nipple. The psychological benefits resulting from these procedures have been demonstrated in many studies, and you should carefully consider the options appropriate for you with your team of care givers.

The simplest approach to restoring a normal profile is with a prosthetic breast worn in your clothing. However, many studies have shown that the psychological trauma are lessened with reconstructive surgery to restore the breast. In some cases, when the surgery is less severe, this can be done simultaneously with the resection, but often it is necessary to wait for a few weeks.

There are several different options for restoring the breast, which vary with your physical condition. Silicone or saline implants, which are receiving much bad publicity recently, can create a proper breast profile in many women. For small breasts, a single insertion will suffice. Large breasts require the skin to stretch, which is done by inserting an inflatable implant that gradually expands to restore the full profile.

The latissimus flap technique (LATS) removes a portion of a muscle in your back and some skin to create part of the breast mound. This leaves an additional scar in the back, but produces a more realistic breast profile.

Transverse rectus abdominus mycocutaneous flap technique (TRAM). This uses a portion of the abdominal muscle and some abdominal fat to restore the breast mound. It has some advantages over the LATS procedure, but also has drawbacks.

The point is there are many options available to restore your physique to near normal. Consult your team of care givers to find out more about them.

SEX

Once, when Bertrand Russell sought medical help for an injury, his doctor asked where it hurt. "In my mind, of course." was his answer.

This story reminds us that we really experience all things in our minds, even tactile sensations. Only when the signal reaches the brain is it placed in the context of everything else going on around us and we formulate a response.

What effect will cancer have on your sex life? The answer is in your mind. Each of us has their individual sensitivity about our sexual appetites, the source of that delicious heterogeneity of our species. Each of us explores and controls them in our unique pattern.

A large part of the sexual experience is tactile, and that may change from the physical differences that follow cancer treatment. Having been through cancer therapy, you will never look at the world quite the same again, and the mental effects on you and your partner are just as significant as any physical changes.

Sexuality is a partnership, and, for different reasons, the following applies to both partners.

There is a period during which many people simply do not feel interested. This can be for physical as well as psychological reasons. Surgery, radiation and chemotherapy all may contribute to physical reactions that make sex uncomfortable, or even painful.

This is followed by a period of anxiety, about pain, about the psychological impact of physical changes in your body, and about the physiological changes that result from treatment. How long each of these periods last is a personal experience.

Counseling and support from your partner can be very helpful. Sometimes there are special anxieties about intercourse, and it may be best to limit contact to less threatening physical expressions of affection while both partners adjust to the new situation.

Many couples have difficulty at first, but there is no reason why the outcome can't be mutually satisfactory. It depends on you and your partner.

HYPERCALCEMIA

Your body is constantly balancing many complex signals to preserve and maintain your health. Often these systems are like thermostats, with signal molecules provoking a series of responses if there is too much "heat," and another set if there is too much "cooling." While your body temperature is one of these carefully maintained balances, there are many others; the thermostat example is meant as a familiar analogy.

One of the most sensitive and interesting is the system for maintaining calcium levels in the blood. The biggest reservoir of calcium is in your skeleton, where 99% of your body's calcium salts make up the bone. Cells within the bones are constantly laying down new and absorbing old bone. Many people are unaware just how often bone matter is replaced (remodeled is the technical word). Ordinarily the uptake and depositing exactly balance.

Calcium comes into your body when it is absorbed by the digestive system, and leaves when excreted by the kidneys, so the main signal system is between these uptake, storage and elimination centers.

Calcium absorbed from bone enters the blood, which distributes it to all the organs. Similarly, if the "thermostat" signals cells to make new bone, blood calcium levels drop.

But calcium plays an important role in controlling many organs and cells, so it is vital to keep the amount of calcium in your blood within the normal range. If the amount gets too high or too low, it can kill you very quickly.

The complexity of the signal system is highly sophisticated, interacting with all the other signal systems of the body. To give you some idea of how it all fits together: we are pretty sure we have identified 30 different signal molecules that can cause bone to be absorbed or produced, we haven't found all of them.

The major hormones whose actions directly affect calcium levels in the blood are: parathyroid hormone, calcitrol (derived from vitamin D), and calcitonin. These interact to control uptake from the gut, elimination through the kidney, and absorption and deposition in the bone. The level of each of these three hormones in the blood is affected by a constellation of signals that are too complex to detail here.

In advanced cancer, one of the burdens placed on your body is to maintain this calcium balance in the face of tumors whose presence throws off all sorts of confusing signals that interrupt the thermostats that regulate things. In some patients, especially in advanced disease, this careful balance can become displaced, and produce too much calcium in the blood (hypercalcemia). This situation can become life threatening very quickly once the balance is disturbed.

The types of cancer that most often lead to hypercalcemia are: breast, multiple myeloma, squamous cell cancer of the lung, and squamous cell head and neck cancer. Other, rarer types of cancer may also increase the amount of calcium in the blood.

It is easy to confuse the effects of hypercalcemia with other influences, such as drug effects or state of disease. One obvious effect of bone loss is how easy it is to break bones. But there are other effects of excess calcium. These include neurologic effects, such as depression, confusion, deafness, and even personality changes. Some effects on the digestive system may be due to calcium imbalance, like vomiting, and/or constipation. The heart may respond with irregular beats, and other effects that would be seen on an electrocardiogram. It can stop the heart dead. The kidneys, too, may be affected, causing an increase in how much urine is produced, which causes dehydration.

What Can Be Done About It?

There are several drugs that can be used to manage hypercalcemia. One factor that must be considered is whether it is worthwhile to treat it at all, given the specific setting.

Hypercalcemia is often a sign that your disease is so advanced that things are seriously going wrong with your body. People generally don't live more than a year after first showing signs of hypercalcemia, and many die within months. If the disease has advanced too far, it may be best not to treat.

Hypercalcemia is diagnosed through changes in the frequency of voiding urine (diuresis), which causes a loss of fluid. This can be treated by giving saline solutions intravenously to boost the fluid volume and increase the flow through the kidneys. This will temporarily restore the proper balance of calcium in the blood. It may be necessary to adjust the concentration of other electrolytes, like potassium and magnesium, as well.

Medications that are used to help your body balance the amount of calcium in your blood include Calcitonin, Glucocorticoids (Prednisone, Dexamethasone or Hydrocortisone), Gallium Nitrate and Bisphosphonates (Pamidronate, Etridonate or Clodronate).

Each of these is effective, but only for a short period. A complex control network like the one that controls calcium balance is difficult to adjust because each change invokes a whole series of responses which try to restore the previous state.

6

CELL BIOLOGY: THE ROOT OF THE DISEASE

WHAT ARE CELLS?

The cell is the basic building block of living things. The cell has a membrane, a kind of skin, around it. Inside is the molecular machinery that gives it life. That is, enables it to make new machinery, turn food into energy, move, reproduce itself and communicate with other cells. Some of these components are arranged in compartments, such as mitochondria, which specialize in producing energy, and the nucleus, which contains the machinery of memory.

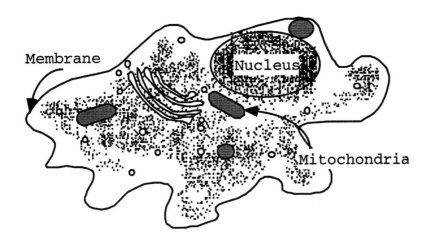

Each of us was once but a single cell. That fertilized ovum reproduced to form two cells, which reproduced again and, through repeated cycles of proliferation, produced a ball containing thousands of cells. At a certain stage in the growth of this ball, the cells started to differ from one another. Those which were the forerunners of the nervous system became slightly, then much, different from those who would make up the digestive system. As this differentiation progressed, the embryo formed that would eventually transform into a human being, made up of trillions of descendants of that first cell.

While all cells share certain common features, there are many degrees of differentiation. A mature liver cell (hepatocyte) bears little resemblance to a muscle or hair follicle cell. That is not surprising, since their jobs are so different.

You can think of differentiation as a family tree, along which are limbs, branching from the different stages of maturation. Near the trunk, very immature liver cells are barely different from very immature muscle cells.

The first steps in differentiation are imperceptible. They could only be detected by going inside the cell to see that the pattern of enzymes and other machinery being produced is slightly different. Gradually, enough material is produced that we can see differences in shape and behavior emerging. At the end of the differentiation pathway there are only traces of similarity between some cell types.

But other cells are more closely related, and have a common ancestor that is only a few generations removed from the end of their pathway. We would represent this by showing their individual branches converging at the point of their common ancestor.

STEM CELLS: MULTIPOTENT REPLACEMENTS

Many of your organs contain immature cells which can be recruited to replace aging or injured cells that are casualties of living. These immature cells can be called upon to form one of several cell types, depending on the need. They are called stem cells, to reflect the fact they are closer to the trunk. There are a few tissues, such as the nervous system, which cannot replace their cells, but most can.

The Path from Original Stem Cell to End Stage Cells

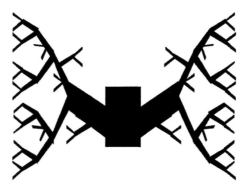

There is enormous diversity in the shape and function of different cells, but their ancestry can all be traced back to that fertilized ovum. As they differentiate, cells take on more and more characteristics of the cell which they are becoming. As they mature, they gradually lose the capacity to reproduce. Most cells at the end of their differentiation pathway can no longer replicate themselves. Partially mature cells can reproduce a few times, while the pluripotent stem cells have almost unlimited capacity to multiply.

Maturation appears as a continuous process, but we know that cells sometimes turn off at key rest stops along the way. They may simply rest, having traveled part way down a maturation pathway, where they await a signal telling them which direction to take next. Or they may reenter the cell cycle again without maturing, which produces a stock of cells who can quickly be recruited as replacements.

As far as we know, once cells start to mature down one of the pathways, they are committed to that path. They cannot back up to become anything other than the cells further along that branch.

These two cell functions: replication, and differentiation plus controlled suicide, are the keys to understanding both normal and abnormal growth. Confusion in the biological signals that regulate these functions is the basis of cancer.

GROWTH CONTROL SIGNALS

Your body is comprised of trillions of cells. Some types of cells are designed for replacement as often as once a day, others are never replaced.

One example of the former are the circulating white blood cells, called neutrophils, which only live a day or so. In order to maintain a constant supply of neutrophils, new ones have to be produced as frequently as the old ones die.

In the marrow of your bones, there is a supply of blood stem cells that can mature to become neutrophils. To maintain an even balance, for each replacement, the stem cell has to reproduce, so one daughter can mature.

This replacement process is highly regulated. There are molecules signaling to hasten replacement, while others tell it to slow down. This balance is one example of a growth control mechanism.

Growth Factor Receptor in Membrane

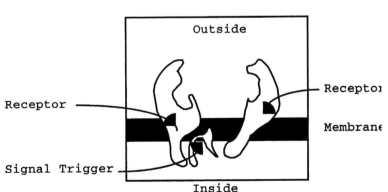

There are many others. When your skin is cut, the platelets that form the clot also give off a growth factor that causes nearby fibroblast cells to start dividing. The fibroblasts proliferate and lay down the collagen fibers that makes the scar tissue to heal the cut in the skin.

Growth factors work by binding to a very specific receptacle molecule present on the outside of the target cell, like a password, that lets the cell know the message is genuine. The signal molecule and its receptor act like a lock and key; only the right shape key can open the lock. Once the receptor molecule is grabbed by the growth factor, it in turn signals inside the cell to trigger the machinery of the cell to begin growing.

Growth Factor Binds to Fire Trigger

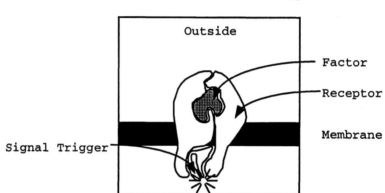

All the molecules involved in this process, including the receptor plus all of the machinery inside the cell that has to perform in order for the cell to multiply, are growth control signals. We don't know exactly how many there are, or what each of them does, but we are learning more and more.

A number of these molecules are associated with various kinds of cancer when they don't function properly. For example, suppose a point mutation cut off one end of a growth factor receptor, so the cell only produced half the molecule. What if the piece made was the half that signals inside the cell? This mutant receptor would constantly be signaling to reproduce because the control part, to which the growth factor is supposed to bind, isn't even there.

Another control mechanism regulates how long a cell lives. If neutrophils are designed to live for 24 hours, what kills them? We're not sure how it works, but we know that cells have a "suicide" bomb inside them which, when activated, kills them, a process called apoptosis. It sounds odd at first, but making sure cells die at the right time is vital.

Apoptosis is controlled by various signal molecules. One form of genetic damage could change the way these controls operate, like a skip in a record that repeats the same sound over and over. The result would be there is too much of one of the signals.

Another type of change could be a point mutation that affects the ability of one of the control molecules to bind to its partner. This, too, could affect cell growth.

HOW CELLS GROW: THE CELL CYCLE

When growing as fast as it can, one of your cells can reproduce every 24 hours. It takes that long to duplicate all the internal components. The process is highly synchronous, and we have a fair understanding of what goes on during each phase of the cycle.

Reproduction

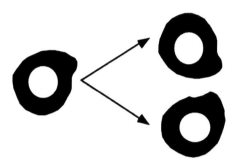

At the beginning, our typical cell has just separated from its sister, and is ready to start the next cycle. The <u>chromosomes</u> unravel, relaxing the DNA package somewhat, in a different structure, called chromatin, that allows better access to the information. Meantime a membrane forms around the chromatin. This partitions the nucleus, containing the chromatin, from the rest of the cell, called the cytoplasm.

The Cell Cycle

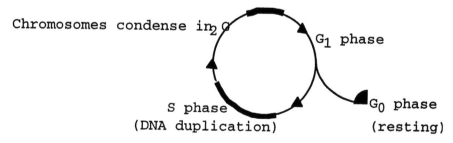

Actual separation into two in M phase

Chromosomes condense in G_2

G_1 phase

S phase
(DNA duplication)

G_0 phase
(resting)

As soon as the nuclear membrane forms, the machinery of the cell starts demanding that new proteins and enzymes be made to carry out the various maintenance activities that go along with being a cell and get ready to divide again. This period of activity is termed G1, the first slice of the cell cycle.

During G1 the cell has one copy each of the DNA bestowed on you by your mother and father. G1 lasts for about 10 hours in a rapidly growing cell.

At the completion of G1, when everything is ready, the cell starts to copy all of its DNA in the next sector of the cycle, called S phase. S (for DNA synthesis) lasts about 6 hours, and is a period of intense synthetic activity.

Once the duplication of the DNA is complete, the cell now has two complete copies of your genetic material, and is said to be in G2 phase. Despite the increase in mass, cells in G2 are metabolizing normally, save the activities that go on in preparation for the actual division.

During G2 the chromatin begins winding itself into tighter and tighter supercoils. This process of condensation is a remarkable feat of packing, when you consider the length of DNA crammed into those minute packets called chromosomes. The cell is entering the last phase, M, as it begins mitosis.

Toward the end of G2, the cell rounds up into a sphere, and the nuclear membrane dissolves. At the end of its condensation, the DNA is wrapped in 92 chromosomes. Two identical sets of chromosomes, one set containing your maternal, the other your paternal inheritance.

The chromosomes align themselves in pairs along the midriff of the cell paired with its twin, so that each half of the cell will have a complete set. The cell apparatus to which the chromosomes attach is called the spindle, so named for the way it looks in a microscope.

Simplified Picture of Chromosomes Align During Mitosis

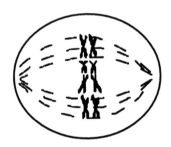

Once the alignment is complete, the pairs of chromosomes are pulled by the machinery of the spindle such that they separate and migrate to the centers of what will be the daughter cells.

Lastly the midriff of the cell begins to contract as if there was a noose around it, pinching the sphere into two daughter cells. M phase only takes about an hour.

Cell Cycle Provides Attack Points for Therapy

When cells reach the final stages of maturation they stop growing and leave the cell cycle. We call this phase G0. Nearly all your cells, whether muscles or kidney or brain, play their piece in the complex symphony of life in this resting phase, G0. This means that the growing cells in G1 are indistinguishable from all the other cells in your body.

But cells in other phases of the cell cycle are performing activities different from resting cells, which are potential attack points. The treatments we use to treat cancer are directed toward killing cells that are carrying out these specific actions.

For example growing cells are the only ones synthesizing DNA, so S phase is a particular target of both anti-cancer drugs and radiotherapy.

M phase is also unique to cells which are dividing, and it is another target of agents designed to kill cancer cells.

The details of how we design agents to attack these points in the cell cycle are given in the section describing the specific anti-cancer drugs and how they work.

How Cells Die: Apoptosis

We are beginning to appreciate that cell death is just as important as producing new cells for the body to function well. If cells fail to die at the right time, they can seriously disturb the balance of signals that make us healthy.

We have discovered cells have a built in device that kills them under the appropriate circumstances. We don't know all the details of the mechanism, but we do know that two proteins are involved, which bind to each other, like the yin/yang symbol.

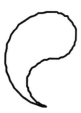 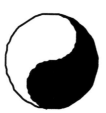 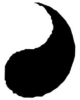

Normally, the two halves are present in equal numbers, and there is harmony. But, when there is an excess of one of these proteins, it may find another partner, and that can unbalance things

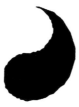

If there is excess yang, it binds to elements in the nucleus that effectively pulls the trigger on the self destruct mechanism. We believe this mechanism is part of the design, and the control of the production of yin and yang can provoke a cell to die if that is

what's needed. For example, during embryonic development, some cells must die to create a space so other cells' growth can make a fold in an newly forming organ.

We are just now learning the importance of this suicide trigger, called apoptosis, in cancer. We believe that some of the drugs used in anti-cancer chemotherapy may work by artificially manipulating the yin:yang balance. As we learn more about the way these elements combine, it may help us design better drugs in the future.

If there is excess yin, it can also present a problem. Cells that have mutated such that they amplify the amount of yin are much, much harder to kill. These cells are able to grow in the presence of many anti-cancer drugs, or radiation or other trauma that would kill normal cells. This means that cells normally are quick to pull the trigger when something's wrong, but too much yin stops the trigger from working.

The real names for yin and yang aren't really important, except to those working on this research. The name for yang is BAX, and yin is bcl-2. p53 is one of the control elements that determines how much yin and yang to make.

WHAT MAKES A CELL MALIGNANT?

We know that tumors arise from a single cell that has failed to respond to the checks and balances that regulate when cells are supposed to multiply and die. When a cell ceases to regulate its growth, a relentless accumulation of the descendants of that cell begins. We believe that accumulated genetic damage (<u>mutation</u>) causes a cell to lose its capacity to respond to either <u>growth control signals</u> or <u>apoptosis</u>. Since the damage is genetic, the daughter cells have inherited this inability to control their growth, and thus the process of tumor formation starts.

Most tumors are benign, meaning the cells multiply locally but are not <u>malignant</u>. Benign tumors appear contained in a kind of capsule, like the yolk in an egg. Benign tumors usually don't change into malignancies, but there are important exceptions, like moles on the skin or intestinal polyps. Your doctor may suggest removing some of these if he feels they may someday risk your health.

Malignancies differ from benign tumors in several ways. For one, they have no defined border, but invade surrounding healthy tissues. They also have more blood vessels, which increase the supply of nourishment to the cells. Inside the cell, the chromosomes are different in appearance, too. Importantly, malignant tumors also differ in the capacity of the cells to break free of the primary tumor and colonize other sites (metastasize).

We are beginning to understand the changes that cells undergo to become malignant. We are certain that the critical events are the accumulated genetic damage to the ancestor of the cells making up the tumor.

However, there are other factors involving how the body responds to the tumor that are equally important in controlling the disease and how it progresses.

To grow, a tumor must induce certain changes. It has to be nourished, for example, which requires new blood vessels form. The production of blood vessels, called angiogenesis, is an important control point in the development of malignancies. Tumors must also alter our immune system, so the white blood cells that cleanse our body of foreign invaders don't recognize and destroy the tumor cells.

Typically breast cancer is diagnosed when a lump is detected during an examination or by mammography. The remarkable success in improving the number of survivors of breast cancer is largely due to the public awareness campaign that has influenced women to examine themselves to catch tumors early. Because of this campaign, breast cancer is usually caught when the tumor is small, and there is a good chance it can be cured.

We usually don't know whether it took ten years or six weeks for a tumor to reach the size where it is detected. Often, most of the growth of a tumor has taken place by the time it its presence is known, and this can present problems for treatment.

CHROMOSOMES: THE GENETIC LIBRARY

Each cell contains a design library for making a new you. This information is in the form of a molecule, called DNA. It works like a videotape, which stores the information to produce a movie when read by the proper machinery[45]. The DNA molecules, like a videotape, are very long, and are wound up in 23 "spools" called chromosomes.

Some Chromosomes

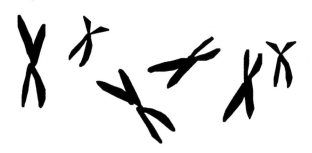

The total length of DNA in one of your cells is over a yard long, yet it is contained inside a cell that is so small it can only be seen using a microscope. This remarkable feat of packaging is done by winding the thread of DNA into coils and winding those coils into supercoils, again and again. The proteins that help wind everything together are called histones.

Think for a moment about the problems that are involved in finding a particular piece of information within the supercoiled DNA, then unwinding the coils and supercoils where that stretch of DNA is buried, so that a copy can be made. This can only happen if something were there that allowed the neighboring coils to relax while the copy is being made. The enzymes whose job is to perform that relaxation are called topoisomerases. These enzymes are important targets of some of the drugs that selectively kill cancer cells.

Except for germ cells, your cells have two sets of "spools," one set from your father, the other from your mother, making 46 chromosomes. (Your germ cells have 23 because they are designed to combine, when fertilized, to produce an ovum that has inherited one set of chromosomes from each parent.)

Incidentally, the number of chromosomes varies between different species. All individuals of that species must have the same number. If they didn't, M phase, where one cell divides the genetic information equally into two daughter cells, would not work. A practical example of this is the mule. A mule is the offspring of two closely related species: a horse mother and a donkey father. Horses and donkeys have different numbers of chromosomes. The two are close enough to produce a healthy offspring, the mule, but the mule cannot produce germ cells because of the unequal division of the chromosomes. So the change in chromosome number is the beginning of separation into two species.

MISTAKES AND MUTATIONS

Each time a cell reproduces, it first makes a complete copy of the DNA, so there will be two to divide between the daughter cells. At the time of separation (M phase), the chromosomes line up in pairs, each with its mate, to make sure the genetic library is equally distributed. When division starts, the pairs are pulled in opposite directions. Then, when the middle of the cell pinches in two to separate the daughter cells, each daughter has a complete set of chromosomes.

Every once in a while, during copying, mistakes happen. Like copying manuscripts, occasionally letters get interchanged, or a period appears in the wrong place. These types of mistakes are called point mutations. Most mutations have little effect, but some can be serious. For example, if a period happens in the middle of a word, it makes a partial word. Usually the partial word is nonsensical and is ignored, but sometimes it can be devastating.

Another kind of mistake happens when two pieces of DNA get rearranged, like skipping a line when reading a book. Two sentences get spliced together, and no longer make sense. Sometimes the new sentence has disastrous consequences. Moving around of the genetic information is called translocation. Genetic translocations can be local rearrangements, or they can involve swapping a whole arm of a chromosome.

Sometimes a piece of DNA gets copied over and over, so a gene might have 50 copies instead of two. Cells can amplify genes intentionally, to be able to produce large amounts of some protein(s) quickly. However, if the wrong gene gets translocated to one of these amplifiers, it could also have serious consequences.

Point mutations and translocations modify the genetic information. Usually the result is unimportant. Sometimes it is harmless, or simply fatal to the cell, which dies as a result. Occasionally it produces a mixed up gene product that affects the whole body.

Once it happens, there is no way to reconstruct the correct information, and if the cell lives, the mistake persists as long as the body. Unless the error happens to be in the germ cells (the cells that unite to conceive a new embryo), mutations and translocations cannot pass on to someone else. These are called somatic mutations, to distinguish them from hereditary mutations, which get passed from one generation to the next.

GENETIC PROBES

The explosion of genetic information that has become available since the introduction of recombinant DNA techniques has made it possible to make probes that tell us whether a specific piece of genetic information is present in a specimen, and how many copies there are.

These probes are used to detect genetic changes in tissue samples. Genetic changes that cause cancer are called oncogenes, and scientists are cataloging them to try and find which ones are going to be useful for telling us how to treat different types of cancer.

Until we have much more information, these different probes aren't used for making decisions about treatment by most physicians. But we are learning quickly, and someday we may be able to use this kind of information to design different treatments, depending on which genetic rearrangement is responsible for an individual patient's disease.

This is the frontier of cancer research. We don't know, yet, how to use this information to design new therapies, but you may be interested in learning our progress in revealing what causes cancer. In many clinical trials one or more of these markers are being tested, to learn more about how they operate in patients (as opposed to research laboratories). You may hear some of these bizarre terms discussed.

HER-2/neu Growth Factor Receptor

HER-2/neu (sometimes called c-erbB-2) is an oncogene that is a mutated form of a normal cell protein. We believe it is a portion of the cell surface receptor to which one of the growth factors binds. In its mutated form, it constantly signals the cell to reproduce, whether the growth factor is present or not.

ras Intracellular Communication Link

Once a signal molecule, such as a growth factor, binds to its receptor, the receptor transfers that message to a number of sites inside the cell. The details of how the message is passed around are complex, but ras is the name of a gene that produces one of the intermediaries, called G protein. Mutations in ras are found in a number of different forms of cancer. Mutant forms of the protein indiscriminately transmit signal to grow.

myc Nuclear Signal Molecules

myc is a gene that codes for a protein that carries signals to the DNA in the nucleus of cells. When it is functioning normally, the myc protein only lives a short while. This means that its digestion is part of the control mechanism; it is produced, delivers its message, then is chewed up, to end the signal. Some mutations produce too much myc protein, and the signal stays "on" all the time. The myc protein is not usually changed by this mutation, but the gene has somehow been amplified many times over.

BCL-2 Control of Cell Death

bcl-2 is a gene that was originally found in a type of lymphoma, and has since been implicated in a number of types of cancer, including prostate, colon, stomach, kidney, lung and brain. It is a gene that is involved in the regulation of cell death (apoptosis). When the bcl-2 gene has been translocated or is produced indiscriminately, cells become immortal.

p53 Tumor Suppresser

p53 is a protein in the nucleus of cells that is part of the thermostat that controls the production of molecules that regulate cell growth and death. Normally, p53 keeps cells from growing.

If there is a mutation that alters p53, so it cannot bind to its partners, the cell can become locked in a continuous growth cycle. In some cancer cells, mutations in p53 like this have been found. There are other cases where p53 is normal, but a another protein is produced that prevents p53 from binding.

In the laboratory, we can stop some tumor cells from growing just by transferring the gene for p53 using genetic engineering. This is why it is called a tumor suppresser gene.

RB Cell Cycle Control

RB is a gene that normally produces a protein involved in regulating the cell cycle. When mutated, the gene produces a protein that no longer binds to its partner(s). When this happens, it causes the cell to lose control of its growth. The mutant was originally isolated from a tumor of the eye (retinoblastoma), but has been found in many other tumors since then.

Cyclin: Cell Cycle Control

Cyclins A, D1 and E are proteins that pass the signal along to the machinery for running the cell cycle. We are at the early stages of understanding whether one or more cyclins are mutated in some types of cancer.

ABL and BCR

Bcr-Abl is a protein produced when two genes are fused through translocation. It is found in nearly all cases of chronic myelogenous leukemia. The product makes the cells who contain it immortal, and resistant to the normal program that causes cell death.

Telomerase

Telomeres are the tips of chromosomes, and they have a special function in the separation of chromosomes during cell division. Telomerase is the enzyme responsible for making the telomeres. Usually, telomerase is only produced in germ cells, the cells producing sperm or eggs.

We believe chromosomes are endowed with telomeres when the germ cells are produced, and cannot add to them again. Each time they divide, our cells gradually lose a small piece of each telomere. Eventually, when the telomeres get too small, the cells can no longer reproduce. So the telomeres act as a counter to limit longevity.

Cancer cells, unlike others, produce telomerase, and therefore can synthesize new telomeres. Perhaps this is due to a mutation in the control mechanism for producing telomerase, or a translocation. The ability to produce more telomeres is crucial for cancer cells unlimited capacity to reproduce.

BRCA1 Inherited Cancer

There are a few families whose members develop cancer of the breast or ovaries much more often than normal, i.e. whose disease is hereditary. We believe this is because a mutation developed in a gene in an ancestor's germ cells, and so was inherited by succeeding generations in those families. The scientists who first identified it named the gene BRCA1.

We don't have a clear picture about how genes cause cancer, but every piece of information helps teach us more about this disease. We know that BRCA1 is mutated in about half the families with hereditary breast cancer, so there must be other genes yet to be discovered.

WHAT HAPPENS WHEN TREATMENT FAILS?

In a nutshell, failures happen because some cells escape the treatment. For surgery and radiation, the cause is cells that had spread before the treatment but escaped detection. For chemotherapy we can only observe the results and speculate about the causes. For those of us studying ways to improve cancer treatment this is an intense area of research.

Experience has taught us that the larger the number of malignant cells (sometimes called the tumor burden), the more likely some are to survive. One reason for this is the larger the tumor, the more daughters of the original cell will differ from each other. Shortly after the tumor has started to grow, all the daughter cells are similar. But as it gets larger, or as cells infiltrate other tissues, they are exposed to different conditions, and these may alter the cells' susceptibility to treatment.

The larger the tumor, the more drug it takes to kill the cells[46]. Side effects limit the amount of drug patients can tolerate, which may not be sufficient to eliminate all of the cells. This is why there is so much attention focused on ways of increasing the amount of drug you can tolerate, to try to surpass this threshold.

Some cancer cells may stop growing temporarily, so they aren't sensitive to the drugs directed against growing cells. Some may spread to compartments in the body where the drugs don't reach. For example, many anti-cancer drugs cannot reach the brain, but cancers often spread there.

Different types of cells vary in their susceptibility to different drugs. We are not sure why this is, but we know that colon and pancreatic cancer responds very poorly to chemotherapy, while breast cancer cells are sensitive to many drugs. Natural resistance is the term used to describe cells that are inherently insensitive to drugs.

Relapses after a period of remission are common. Some patients go through many cycles of remission and relapse, while others fail rapidly when the disease returns.

We know that a few cells exposed to chemotherapy adapt, such that they are much less susceptible to the drug. This phenomenon is called acquired resistance. Cells that have acquired resistance are very difficult to kill because they become resistant to many drugs when this happens, not just the drugs to which they have been exposed.

One form of acquired resistance that has been studied extensively is the multi-drug resistance (MDR) phenomenon. We have learned through MDR how the cell machinery changes to decrease their susceptibility to cytotoxic drugs. This information has been used to try and subvert this mechanism with drugs designed to block the MDR machinery.

It is likely that other mechanisms yet to be discovered can also confer resistance, as life constantly adapts to change.

The dynamics of the interactions between our body's complex network of control systems and its response to cancer is the subject of a lot of research. When the body's control systems are exhausted, a relapse can be devastating. Some of the tools of this control network are known, and make up the armory of biological therapy, but some have yet to be discovered.

It may be cold comfort, but the learning process is slow. It is one thing to identify the array of biological signals involved in fighting cancer, but the knowledge of how to combine them to effectively fight this disease is only emerging slowly.

MULTI-DRUG RESISTANCE

When we expose tumor cells in the laboratory to low doses of anti-cancer drugs, two things can happen. Many cells get very sick and die, but a few continue to live. These cells have acquired the ability to grow in the presence of this drug, and are said to be resistant[47].

We also observe that cells which have acquired resistance have also become resistant to a whole battery of anti-cancer drugs, many of which appear totally unrelated to each other. These cells are said to have acquired multi-drug resistance (MDR).

Study of the machinery of MDR+ cells has shown us that they have a pump embedded in the membrane on their surface. This pump is a protein that has sugar molecules bound to it (which makes it a glycoprotein), and has a molecular weight of about 170,000. It is often called the P-glycoprotein, or GP170.

This protein literally pumps cytotoxic drugs out of the cell very rapidly. As a result, cells with the P-glycoprotein, when bathed in a solution containing a drug, have far less of the drug inside than sensitive cells. They are able to grow because the drug doesn't stay inside the cells.

Once this P-glycoprotein was found and characterized, researchers looked to see whether it could be identified in tumors from patients who were treated with chemotherapy. It has been found on cells that are naturally resistant, such as colon cancer cells, and it is found on cells from patients that have relapsed because their tumors have become resistant.

MDR is not the only mechanism by which tumors become resistant, but it is one significant clue in developing the complete picture.

7

Putting It All Together

You feel bewildered by all of the different facets of this disease. Perhaps it will help put everything in perspective to look over the process of diagnosis and treatment again.

The disease is caused by a series of genetic mutations that caused one cell to reproduce uncontrollably. That cell and its daughters have been growing long enough to produce a tumor. How serious that is depends on how long its been growing and where.

If caught early, breast cancer is curable. If it has metastasized, it must be removed by a combination of surgery, radiation and chemotherapy. Treatment of advanced disease is successful in thousands of cases, but not as often as we would like. We do know that, overall, patients who undergo chemotherapy live longer than those who do not.

We don't have enough information about experimental therapies to say for sure which will improve your chances for survival. Patients with Stage III or IV disease should consider these options, which include new drugs, high dose consolidation, or neoadjuvant therapy.

You would be helping other patients and the community of people trying to design treatments if you did this in a clinical trial. If you did, your case could be pooled with others to provide statistics to help us analyze how successful the treatment is. However, you should know that you can receive treatment without joining a clinical trial (except drugs that have not yet been approved by the FDA).

Treatment of advanced disease is usually successful at reducing or eliminating the tumor and killing many metastases. However, it is not uncommon for pockets to return after a period of remission. Patients who experienced a significant improvement from chemotherapy are likely to respond well to further treatment. Often cycles of remission and relapse can control the disease for many years, even decades.

If you have successfully been treated with traditional chemotherapy but relapsed, you may wish to consider high dose chemotherapy with stem cell support, such as bone marrow transplant, as the next stage of treatment. The statistics are not available, but there is a strong feeling in the community that this is likely to be the treatment of choice when they are.

Researchers are learning a lot about the changes in the cell that produced the tumor. We don't yet have enough information to make the explanation simple. Many groups are approaching the problem from different angles, and we don't know how they will converge in a consistent story.

You have read about some of the molecular systems that interact to produce this loss of growth control, like apopotosis, telomerases, or mutated growth factor receptors. This isn't necessary information, but may help satisfy your curiosity about what is being done to develop new treatments for the future.

The more you know about the disease, the better prepared you will be to participate in the fight against this disease, and become a partner in the design of your therapy.

APPENDICES

DRUGS USED IN CHEMOTHERAPY

The following comprehensive list is provided to give you some information about drugs you might encounter in the treatment of cancer. It includes some experimental drugs, but not all. The purpose is so you can look up the different types of drugs, and help you understand the plan underlying a suggested course of therapy.

It also provides some history of the associated side effects that have been found in testing these drugs. Obviously, there are many factors that will impact on which of these side effects you might experience, including your age, the state of health of your different organ systems, the dose you are receiving and the impact of your disease. You can take measures to control some of these side effects, and these measures are discussed a previous section.

Allopurinol

Allopurinol, also known as Zyloprim, is not an anti-cancer agent, but a drug that is used to reduce some of the side effects of cancer therapy.

It is a synthetic compound designed to block the enzyme xanthine oxidase. This enzyme is involved in the body's mechanism for the elimination of nitrogen through the production of uric acid. It is used to treat conditions where uric acid accumulation is a problem, such as gout. Patients who have a very large number of cancer cells have trouble disposing of the cellular debris after these cells are killed by intensive radiation and/or chemotherapy. Allopurinol helps control this problem by managing the production of uric acid during elimination of some of the products of that debris.

Allopurinol is taken orally.

- Severe rash may develop in 2% of the patients taking allupurinol, but generally the toxicity is not a problem.

Altretamine

Altretamine, also known as Hexamethylmelamine, or Hexalen® (US Bioscience), is a synthetic compound recently approved by the FDA. It has been known for many years that Altretamine is an active anti-cancer drug, but the proportion of patients who responded in human clinical trials was low. More recently, however, clinical trials in patients with renal cell carcinoma and ovarian cancer that didn't respond to standard therapies, did show a response to Altretamine.

Altretamine is similar to a class of drugs called alklylating agents, along with Ifosfamide and Procarbazine. We believe alkylating agents work by binding to the DNA and causing problems with its duplication. However, when tested against cells in the laboratory, Altretamine doesn't appear to act as an alkyllator. Either it works by a different mechanism, or it works differently in the body than it does in the laboratory.

Altretamine is given orally as a capsule.

SIDE EFFECTS

- Gastrointestinal toxicity is the primary side effect of Altretamine therapy. This takes the form of weight loss, nausea, vomiting, diarrhea and cramps.
- Peripheral neural toxicity is also common. This might show up as numbness, loss of tendon reflexes, loss of coordination (ataxia) or tingling, such as you get when you bump your "funny bone" (paresthesia).
- Central neural toxicity can show up as agitation, confusion, hallucinations, depression, or involuntary shaking. These effects disappear after a while.
- Bone marrow toxicity (myelosuppression) is usually mild.
- Hair loss, skin rash, and temporary rises of levels in the blood of substances that indicate kidney and liver toxicities are sometimes observed, too.

Aminoglutethimide

Aminoglutethimide, also known as Cytadren, Elipten or Orimeten, is a synthetic product. It is not an anti-cancer drug, but blocks some enzymes which helps control the side effects caused by certain cancers.

Some patients with breast or prostate cancer develop a glandular disorder known as Cushing's syndrome. There are multiple symptoms to this syndrome, some of which are:

eight gain due to fluid retention, acne, high blood pressure and mental illness. This effect is due to an imbalance in the secretion of certain hormones in the adrenal cortex, in reaction to cancer. Combined with Hydrocortisone, Aminoglutethimide shuts off the production of steroid hormones (cortisols, estrogen and androgens) by the adrenals, and controls the symptoms.

It is given orally as a tablet.

SIDE EFFECTS

- An allergic skin reaction is seen in more than half the patients who receive Aminoglutethimide. Usually this goes away in 5 days or so.
- Lethargy, sleepiness and dizziness are not as frequent but can be remarkable in individual patients.

Bisphosphonates

Bisphosphonates are small synthetic molecules designed to mimic the inorganic electrolyte, pyrophosphate. They are not anti-cancer drugs, but are used to control one of the side effects that cancer patients experience in late stage disease, hypercalcemia. There are three commonly used Bisphosphonates, Etridonate (Didronel®), Clodronate and Pamidronate (Aredia®). They are all different, but are grouped here for convenience.

Pyrophosphates are produced as part of many biochemical processes. Among their biological roles, is to affect osteoclasts, the cells responsible for resorbing bone. As a result, Bisphosphonates reduce bone resorption and tip the balance controlling blood calcium levels toward lowering those levels.

Bisphosphonates are given initially by intravenous infusion over a few hours. Oral forms of Pamidronate and Clodronate are also available for daily use.

SIDE EFFECTS

- Bisphosphonates are well tolerated, although there is always a risk of damage to the kidneys.
- Chronic use may eventually cause symptoms such as stomach ache, which can evolve into serious problems with the digestive system.

Bleomycin

Bleomycin, also known by its brand name Blenoxane® (Bristol-Myers Oncology) is an antibiotic originally discovered in soil samples. Bacteria living in soil have evolved ways to produce many noxious compounds to help them compete with other bacteria that share their habitat. Pharmaceutical companies have been systematically collecting soil samples from around the world for years, and many of our most important antibiotics have come from different members of a bacterial family called Streptomyces.

Bleomycin is actually a mixture of small peptides purified from bacteria grown in fermentation vats. The peptides are complexed with metal ions, which they carry into the cell's DNA. Once activated, the Bleomycin:metal complex causes multiple breaks in the cell chromosomes, which are then prevented from replicating. Bleomycin works during a specific part of the cell cycle, G2 phase.

Bleomycin is an active anti-cancer agent and is used in a number of diseases, including cancers of the lung, head and neck, cervix, skin, vagina, penis, testicles, rectum, as well as different types of lymphoma. It is a component of many combination therapies because it does not cause bone marrow toxicity.

Bleomycin is given by injection, either into a muscle, under the skin, or directly into a vein.

SIDE EFFECTS

- Fever, sometimes with chills, happens to half the patients who receive Bleomycin.
- Skin reactions are quite common with Bleomycin therapy. These run from reddening of the skin, increased pigmentation, to swelling (edema) and irritation of the mucous membranes (stomatitis).
- Hair loss is a frequent side effect, but usually reverses. Hair loss (called alopecia) does not threaten your health, but it can have a profound affect on how you feel about yourself.
- Many patients find the changes to their appearance, such as alopecia or changes in their fingernails, more devastating than the events that are more significant from a medical point of view.
- Lung damage, which doesn't show up for some time after dosing, is a common and serious side effect. Bleomycin affects the cells in the lung, and this effect may be enhanced in older patients and in patients whose lungs are treated with radiotherapy. Though rarely, this lung toxicity can be fatal.

Busulfan

Busulfan, also known as Busulphan, BSF or by its brand name Myerlan® (Burroughs Wellcome) is a drug in the nitrogen mustard family, related to Chlorambucil and Cyclophosphamide. These compounds were originally discovered for chemical warfare during World War I. The first drugs used in anti-cancer chemotherapy were nitrogen mustards.

All the nitrogen mustard drugs convert to an active species after they get inside a cell. Once activated, they are highly interactive with a number of different molecules, but the most important target is the cell's chromosomes. They bind to DNA and crosslink the strands (called alkylation), which prevents DNA from being duplicated, and either kills the cell or stops it from dividing. The various nitrogen mustards differ in potency, toxicity and what kind of tumors they are active against. We believe the differences result from the rate they get into various cells, how quickly they convert, and what kind of damage they inflict once there.

Busulfan is effective against certain leukemias and is used to promote stem cell growth in bone marrow transplantation.

Busulfan is given orally as a tablet.

SIDE EFFECTS

- Bone marrow toxicity (myelosuppression) is observed at high doses of Busulfan. This is a side effect of killing the stem cells in your bone marrow that produce new blood cells. This toxicity is detected when the cells in your blood are counted. The laboratory typically finds a reduction in white cells (neutropenia) and platelets (thrombocytopenia). The lowest counts are usually 11 to 30 days after the drug was given. Bone marrow toxicity is temporary, since not all the stem cells are killed, and your white cell counts will return to normal 30 to 50 days after the drug is given.
- Lung damage is a well documented problem with high doses of Busulfan therapy. It may take years to develop, but is often fatal when it occurs.
- Nausea and vomiting are not normal in low dose Busulfan therapy, but will evolve at higher doses. Diarrhea is sometimes experienced, too.
- Skin effects include increased pigmentation.

Calcitonin

Calcitonin is not an anti-cancer drug, but is used to help control one of the side effects of cancer, hypercalcemia. It is a short peptide hormone that your body's cells normally produce to help maintain the right amount of calcium in your blood. Commercial sources of Calcitonin are purified from human tissues (Cibacalcin® sold by Novartis), salmon (Miacalcin® from Novartis) or synthetic (Calcimar® from Rhone-Poulenc Rohrer).

Calcitonin is given by injection into a muscle.

SIDE EFFECTS

- Nausea is experienced by many people shortly after injection, but is not serious.
- Mild flushing of the skin, stomach cramps also are reported, but generally Calcitonin is well tolerated.
- A few people experience an allergic reaction.

Carboplatin

Carboplatin, also known by Bristol-Myers Oncology's brand name of Paraplatin®, is a recently approved, synthetic compound in the platinum family, designed to be more effective than Cisplatin. In comparison studies, Carboplatin was similar or slightly better than Cisplatin for some types of cancer. It has been tested most thoroughly in treatment of Ovarian cancer, but it has also shown activity in other diseases, including cancers of the lung, cervix, bladder, testes, head and neck and certain brain tumors. It is not active against tumors that have become resistant to Cisplatin.

Carboplatin probably works by binding to DNA, similar to Cisplatin, although the mechanism is not completely understood. We believe that Carboplatin is not the active form of the molecule, but that it converts to the active form after it gets into the cell. Where and when this conversion takes place affects its ability to kill tumor cells and also is responsible for its toxicity. It is likely that the differences between Cisplatin and Carboplatin are related to how fast they convert and where the conversion takes place. Both compounds create crosslinks between DNA, although the rates at which these appear differ.

Carboplatin is given by injection into a vein over at least 15 minutes.

SIDE EFFECTS

- Toxicity to the Bone marrow (myelosuppression) is the side effect that poses the most significant problem with Carboplatin. This contrasts with Cisplatin, which rarely causes myelosuppression.
- Myelosuppression results from killing the stem cells in your bone marrow that produce new blood cells. This toxicity is detected when the cells in your blood are counted. The laboratory typically finds a reduction in white cells (leukopenia) and platelets (thrombocytopenia). The latter is most pronounced with Carboplatin. The lowest platelet counts are usually 21 days after the drug was given. Bone marrow toxicity is temporary, since not all the stem cells are killed, and your white cell counts will return to normal 4 to 5 weeks after the drug is given. If your marrow has already been depleted by previous treatments, this toxicity can be even more severe.
- Nausea and vomiting (emesis) are not as common side effects as with Cisplatin. With combinations of corticosteroids and new anti-emetic drugs, many patients can control emesis with Carboplatin.
- Diarrhea and constipation are side effects that affect some patients.
- Kidney damage (nephrotoxicity) is not as frequent or as severe as is seen with Cisplatin. This is probably because the timing of the conversion of Carboplatin is different. Between 10 and 20% of patients will have some mild nephrotoxicity. Your doctor will detect this from the results of your blood tests, which may show high levels of creatinine, urea nitrogen, uric acid and/or magnesium. A few patients find blood in their urine, a condition which should resolve itself.
- Nerve damage (neurotoxicity) happens to a few percent of patients receiving Carboplatin, especially those who are on large doses. The symptoms reported are: a numbing or tingling sensation. These are less severe symptoms than those in patients who are given Cisplatin.
- Hearing problems are also less severe than are found with Cisplatin. Hearing loss can be measured in some patients, but often reverses after treatment is finished.
- Hair loss, skin problems and mouth sores occur only rarely.

Carmustine (BCNU)

Carmustine is also known as BCNU, bischloronitrosourea, and by its brand name of BiCNU® (Bristol Myers Oncology). It is a synthetic nitrosourea compound, in the same category as Lomustine, and Streptozocin.

It is an alkylating agent, and converts to a short lived, highly reactive molecule, which is the effective compound. Once the molecule is armed, it binds to DNA and proteins, which stops them from functioning and blocks the cell from duplicating.

Carmustine has been used against many types of cancer for thirty years, including lymphomas, myelomas and cancers of the brain, lung, breast and gastrointestinal systems.

It is given by injection into the vein, usually infused over at least 30 minutes, and often longer.

SIDE EFFECTS

- Toxicity to the Bone marrow (myelosuppression) is the most significant side effect with Carmustine. Depletion of the marrow takes longer than with most anti-cancer drugs, and can be severe. Myelosuppression results from killing the stem cells in your bone marrow that produce new blood cells. It is detected when the cells in your blood are counted. The laboratory typically finds a reduction in white cells (neutropenia) and platelets (thrombocytopenia). The lowest white cell and platelet counts are usually seen 3 to 5 weeks after the drug is given. Bone marrow toxicity is temporary, since not all the stem cells are killed, and your white cell counts will return to normal, usually within 4 to 8 weeks after the drug is given. If your marrow has already been depleted by previous treatments, this toxicity can be even more severe.
- Immediate reaction to Carmustine often include pain at the site of injection and flushing of the skin. Carmustine is irritating to the skin, and contact should be avoided.
- Nausea and vomiting (emesis) are very common side effects, and start about 2 hours after the injection. Even with combinations of glucocorticoids and new anti-emetic drugs, many patients still have terrible nausea.
- Kidney and liver damage are sometimes seen with Carmustine therapy. These show up in test results when your blood is analyzed, and usually go away without problems.
- If the dose of Carmustine is very high, damage to the liver and/or kidney can be severe in some patients, due to interrupted blood flow through these organs. This condition can be life threatening.
- Lung damage is seen with intensive Carmustine therapy in some patients. Damage to the lungs can be quite severe, even fatal.

Chlorambucil

Chlorambucil is also known as CB-1348, chloraminophene or by its brand name Leukeran® (Glaxo Wellcome). It is derived from the nitrogen mustard family, which includes Cyclophosphamide and Ifosfamide. These compounds were originally exploited as chemical weapons during World War I. The first drugs used in anti-cancer chemotherapy were nitrogen mustards.

It is an alkylating agent, and converts to a short lived, highly reactive molecule, which is the effective compound. Once the molecule is armed, it binds to DNA and proteins (alkylation), which stops them from functioning and blocks the cell from duplicating. Chlorambucil is one of easiest alkylating agents to tolerate because it converts more slowly than others.

Chlorambucil is active against many types of cancer, including cancers of the blood (leukemia and lymphoma), ovarian and breast cancer. It is often combined with other agents to enhance its activity.

It is given orally, as a tablet.

SIDE EFFECTS

- Toxicity to the Bone marrow (myelosuppression) is the most significant side effect with Chlorambucil. Depletion of the marrow takes longer to appear than with most anti-cancer drugs, but is severe. Permanent damage to the marrow can happen. It is suspected that Chlorambucil can cause leukemia as well as treat it. Myelosuppression results from killing the stem cells in your bone marrow that produce new blood cells. It is detected when the cells in your blood are counted. The laboratory typically finds a reduction in white cells (neutropenia), antibody producing cells (lymphocytopenia) and platelets (thrombocytopenia). The lowest white cell and platelet counts are usually seen 3 to 5 weeks after the drug is given. Bone marrow toxicity is temporary, since not all the stem cells are killed, and your white cell counts will return to normal 4 to 8 weeks after the drug is given. If your marrow has already been depleted by previous treatments, this toxicity can be even more severe.
- Affects on the nervous system are sometimes seen at very high doses. These affects can include seizures and coma.
- Nausea and vomiting (emesis) are common side effects, but can be controlled.
- Skin toxicity, such as rash and swelling happens to some patients.
- Sperm production is affected and Chlorambucil is known to produce birth defects.
- Lung damage has been reported for patients taking Chlorambucil for a long time. While this is usually reversible, it can be fatal.

Cisplatin

Platinol® is Bristol-Myers Oncology's brand name of a simple inorganic molecule that has proven to be one of the most effective drugs against solid tumors. Other names are Cisplatin, DDP, CACP and cis-platinum. It is commonly used in combination with various other anti-cancer drugs, such as VP-16, cyclophosphamide, or vinblastine in the treatment of many types of cancer.

It is not platinum metal, but an inorganic molecule containing platinum. We think it works by binding to DNA after becoming activated inside the cell. We believe that Cisplatin is not the active form of the molecule, but that it becomes activated after it gets into the target cell. Where and when this conversion takes place affects its ability to kill tumor cells and also is responsible for its toxicity. It also binds to different proteins inside the cell, and we're not sure exactly how these different binding events selectively kill tumor cells.

It is active against many solid tumors, including cancers of the testis, penis, ovary, head and neck, bladder, lung, stomach, cervix, prostate, breast, sarcomas, lymphomas and some brain tumors.

Cisplatin is administered by intravenous infusion.

SIDE EFFECTS

- Nausea and vomiting (emesis) are the most common side effects of cisplatin. It is so common and can be so severe that drugs have been developed especially to work on the part of the brain that controls emesis. Combinations of corticosteroids and these anti-emetic drugs controls emesis in most, but not all patients.
- Kidney damage (nephrotoxicity) can be life threatening, and is the most common reason for limiting or stopping the dose. Doctors have learned that giving fluids to increase flow through the kidneys before dosing with platinum helps protect them, so it has become routine practice.
- Hearing loss (ototoxicity) is another common side effect of platinol. The high pitch sounds are lost first, and can happen in one or both ears. Sometimes ear aches are felt. Increasing the amount of fluids in your body just before dosing also helps control hearing loss. It often, but not always, gets better in time.
- Nerve damage. Many patients experience a tingling or numbness in their arms and legs after platinum therapy. There have been cases of more severe problems, such as effects on the brain, but these are rare.
- Bone marrow toxicity (myelosuppression) is sometimes seen with high doses of cisplatin. But it is not usually a problem. This is a side effect of killing the stem cells in your bone marrow that produce new blood cells. This toxicity is detected when the cells in your blood are counted. The laboratory typically finds a reduction in white cells (neutropenia) and platelets (thrombo-cytopenia). The lowest counts are usually 16 days after the drug was given. Bone marrow toxicity is temporary, since not all the stem cells are killed, and your white cell counts will return to normal 22 days after the drug is given.
- Allergic reactions can develop in patients who have received cisplatin treatment in the past. Swelling, wheezing, drop in blood pressure are all symptoms. These side effects can be controlled with drugs like antihistamines or the cortisone family of corticosteroids.

Cladribine

Cladribine is a synthetic molecule designed to imitate a natural component of DNA, adenosine, and short circuit enzymes who work on adenosine. As such it is classified as an antimetabolite, similar to Pentostatin. It is also known as 2-CdA, or by the brand name Leustatin® (Ortho Biotech).

Antimetabolites work best on cells at a particular point (S phase) in the cell cycle, so it is most effective when the dose is given over 24 hours, making sure all of the sensitive cells go through S phase with the drug present.

Cladribine must be activated by the cell in order to be effective, and the rate of conversion affects its effectiveness and its toxicity. It was recently approved by the FDA for use in hairy cell leukemia, and has shown activity against lymphoma.

It is administered by intravenous infusion over 24 hours.

SIDE EFFECTS

- Toxicity to the Bone marrow (myelosuppression) is the most significant side effect with Cladribine. Myelosuppression results from killing the stem cells in your bone marrow that produce new blood cells. It is detected when the cells in your blood are counted. The laboratory typically finds a reduction in white cells (neutropenia), and antibody producing cells (lymphocytopenia). The lowest white cell counts are usually seen 1 to 2 weeks after the drug is given. Bone marrow toxicity is temporary, since not all the stem cells are killed, and your white cell counts will return to normal about 4 weeks after the drug is given. If your marrow has already been depleted by previous treatments, this toxicity can be even more severe.
- Nausea and Vomiting, hair loss or damage to the kidneys or liver are rare.

CPT-11

CPT-11 was recently approved by the FDA. It is produced by modifying a compound that is extracted from a tree found in China. The natural product, Camptothecin, is another in the long list of folk medicines which contain an active compound when analyzed by scientists. Camptothecin proved too toxic when tested in clinical trials, so modifications have been made to the molecule. CPT-11 and Topotecan are both derived from this compound.

Other names are Camptothecin-11, Irinotecan and Camptosar® (Pharmacia and Upjohn). All these compounds work by blocking the topoisomerase enzymes, which prevents the cell from duplicating its chromosomes. It has been studied more in Japan than in the U.S., but used to treat in cervical, colorectal and lung cancer.

It is administered by intravenous infusion.

SIDE EFFECTS

- Toxicity to the Bone marrow (myelosuppression) is the side effect of CPT-11 that is of most concern.
- Nausea and vomiting (emesis).
- Severe diarrhea that cannot be controlled by supportive care is a serious problem that may restrict the use of CPT-11.
- Hair loss is a frequent side effect, but usually reverses. Hair loss (called alopecia) does not threaten your health, but it can have a profound affect on how you feel about yourself.

- Many patients find the changes to their appearance, such as alopecia or changes in their fingernails, more devastating than the events that are more significant from a medical point of view.

Cyclophosphamide

Cyclophosphamide is also known as CTX, Cycloblastin, or by one of its several trade names: Cytoxan® (Bristol-Myers Oncology) Endoxan® (Asta-Werke) or Neosar® (Adria). It is a synthetic member of the nitrogen mustard family, which includes Chlorambucil and Ifosfamide. These compounds were originally exploited for chemical warfare during World War I. The first drugs used in anti-cancer chemotherapy were nitrogen mustards.

All the nitrogen mustard drugs convert to an active species once they get inside a cell. Once converted, they are highly interactive with a number of different molecules, but the most important target is the cell's chromosomes. They bind to DNA and crosslink the strands (called alkylation), which prevents DNA from being duplicated, and either kills the cell or stops it from dividing. The various nitrogen mustards differ in potency, toxicity and what kind of tumors they are active against. The differences are attributed to the rate they get into various cells, how quickly they convert, and what kind of damage they inflict once there.

Cyclophosphamide is effective against many types of cancer, and is often a component of combination chemotherapy. It is used to treat cancers of the lung, breast, testis, prostate, cervix, ovaries, brain, sarcomas, lymphomas, myeloma, endometrium and leukemia. It can be used to mobilize stem cells into the blood prior to stem cell support.

Cyclophosphamide can be given either by intravenous infusion or as an oral tablet.

SIDE EFFECTS

- Bone marrow toxicity (myelosuppression) is the most common side effect of Cyclophosphamide. Myelosuppression results from killing the stem cells in your bone marrow that produce new blood cells. This condition is detected when the cells in your blood are counted. The laboratory typically finds a reduction in white cells (neutropenia) and, less often, platelets (thrombo-cytopenia). The lowest counts are usually seen between day 8 and 14 after the drug was given. Bone marrow toxicity is temporary, since not all the stem cells are killed, and your white cell counts will return to normal 18 to 25 days after the drug is given.
- Bladder damage is another well documented side effect of Cyclophosphamide. Frequently blood is observed in the urine and the condition often leads to cystitis. It may not appear for a day or even a week after treatment, but can be severe. Often you will be hydrated (given lots of fluids) to increase the flow rate through the bladder to control this condition. Mesna is a drug that is frequently given along with Cyclophosphamide to help control bladder damage.
- Bladder cancer has been reported in a few patients who have received Cyclophosphamide therapy.

- Hair loss is a frequent side effect, but usually reverses. Hair loss (called alopecia) does not threaten your health, but it can have a profound affect on how you feel about yourself.
- Many patients find the changes to their appearance, such as alopecia or changes in their fingernails, more devastating than the events that are more significant from a medical point of view.
- Gastrointestinal toxicity, including anorexia, nausea and vomiting is common, especially in patients receiving high doses of Cyclophosphamide.
- Lung damage is sometimes observed in patients taking Cyclophosphamide. This usually results when the drug is given for a long time, and develops slowly. It is serious, and frequently fatal.
- Atrophy of the testicles or interruption of the menstrual cycle are both effects of the drug interrupting production of hormones.

Cytarabine (Ara-C)

Cytarabine is also known as Ara-C, cytosine arabinoside or by the brand name Cytosar-U (Pharmacia and Upjohn). It is a synthetic compound designed to mimic the natural component of DNA, cytosine, and short circuit enzymes who use it.

Cytarabine is classified as an antimetabolite, meaning it affects some of the enzymes used to synthesize or breakdown (metabolize) molecules. Antimetabolites work best on cells at a particular point (S phase) in the cell cycle, so it is most effective when the dose is given over 24 hours, to make sure all of the sensitive cells go through S phase with the drug present.

Cytarabine must be activated by the cell in order to be effective, and the rate of conversion affects its potency and its toxicity. It is active against and often used to treat leukemia, lymphomas and cancer of the head and neck and stomach.

Cytarabine is administered by injection, either as an intravenous infusion or by injection just below the skin (subcutaneous) or into the muscle (intramuscular).

SIDE EFFECTS

- Bone marrow toxicity (myelosuppression) is the most common side effect of Cytarabine. Myelosuppression results from killing the stem cells in your bone marrow that produce new blood cells. It is detected when the cells in your blood are counted. The laboratory typically finds a reduction in white cells (neutropenia). The lowest counts are usually seen between day 15 and 24 after the drug was given. Your white cell counts will return to normal 10 days after this. Platelet reduction (thrombocytopenia) is most severe between 12 and 15 days and returns to normal 10 days later.
- Nausea and vomiting (emesis) are common side effects of Cytarabine. It is so common and can be so severe that drugs have been developed especially to work on the part of the brain that controls emesis. Even with combinations of corticosteroids and these new drugs, many patients still have terrible nausea.
- Other effects on the digestive system include diarrhea and intestinal bleeding.

- Mouth sores (stomatitis) are common and very unpleasant side effects. They are extremely painful, and affect your ability to swallow. It is important to keep your mouth clean and moist until this condition goes away.
- Liver, kidney and pancreas damage has been observed in a few patients, so is considered possible.
- Eye irritation (conjunctivitis) can be a problem, especially with high doses of Cytarabine. Eyedrops containing a drug like dexamethasone help control this. More severe eye toxicity, such as pain, blurred vision and aversion to light happen to some patients. This condition will go away in time.
- Flushing of the skin, and sometimes rashes on the palms, soles of the feet, chest and neck are reported. They may be associated with symptoms like fever, pain in your muscles and bone, and just feeling very sick (malaise).
- Nerve damage, which usually (but doesn't always) go away, is known to happen, especially with large doses. This is detected as lack of muscle coordination, which can be seen in eye movements, in slurred speech, balance or other kinds of movement.
- Cytarabine can cause birth defects.

Dacarbazine (DTIC)

Dacarbazine, also known as DTIC or DIC, is a synthetic compound that works by a different mechanism than it was originally designed to do. It was thought to be an antimetabolite, but we now believe its activity is through interrupting production of DNA by a different chemical pathway.

It is active against several types of cancers, including Hodgkin's lymphoma, melanoma, and sarcomas.

Dacarbazine is given intravenously, either in a short infusion or all at once.

SIDE EFFECTS

- Nausea and vomiting (emesis) are very common side effects of Dacarbazine. Emesis is so common and can be so severe that drugs have been developed especially to control it. Even with combinations of corticosteroids and the new anti-emetic drugs, many patients still have terrible nausea for up to 12 hours after receiving Dacarbazine.
- Bone marrow toxicity (myelosuppression) is a common side effect of Dacarbazine, but is usually mild. Myelosuppression results from killing the stem cells in your bone marrow that produce new blood cells. It is detected when the cells in your blood are counted. The laboratory typically finds a reduction in white cells (neutropenia) and platelets (thrombocytopenia). The lowest counts are usually seen between day 21 and 25 after the drug was given. Your white cell counts will return to normal about 10 days after this.
- Hair loss is a frequent side effect, but usually reverses. Hair loss (called alopecia) does not threaten your health, but it can have a profound affect on how you feel about yourself.
- Many patients find the changes to their appearance, such as alopecia or changes in their fingernails, more devastating than the events that are more significant from a medical point of view.

- Damage to the liver is a known risk of Dacarbazine therapy. This may not show up for a few days, but can be severe, even fatal.
- Flu-like symptoms are often reported, including fever, pain in your muscles and bone, and just feeling very sick (malaise).
- Light sensitivity, including pain on the head and hands when exposed to sunlight, is rare.

Dactinomycin

Dactinomycin is also known as Actinomycin D, ACT-D, ACT or by its brand name of Cosmegen® (Merck). It is an antibiotic originally discovered in soil samples. Bacteria living in soil have evolved ways to produce many noxious compounds to help them compete against other bacteria that share their habitat. Pharmaceutical companies have been systematically collecting soil samples from around the world for years, and many of our most important antibiotics have come from different members of a bacterial family called Streptomyces.

It binds to DNA, causing it to twist and interfering with a number of the enzymes involved in maintaining the supercoil packing of DNA in the cell chromosomes (topoisomerases).

Dactinomycin is active against a number of different tumors, including cancer of the testis, Wilm's tumor, melanoma, choriocarcinoma, neuroblastoma, retinoblastoma and sarcomas.

Dactinomycin is given intravenously by slow infusion.

SIDE EFFECTS

- Dactinomycin causes a severe reaction to tissues it comes in contact with. Great care should be taken to make sure it all goes into the vein at the site of injection. Bone marrow toxicity (myelosuppression) is the most common side effect of Dactinomycin. Myelosuppression results from killing the stem cells in your bone marrow that produce new blood cells. It is detected when the cells in your blood are counted. The laboratory typically finds a reduction in white cells (neutropenia) and platelets (thrombocytopenia). The lowest counts are usually seen 3 weeks after the drug is given. Your white cell counts will return to normal 10 to 14 days after this.
- Dactinomycin used to be used to suppress the immune system after organ transplants. This activity intensifies the risk of infection from bacteria or viruses during the period when your immune system is depleted.
- Nausea and vomiting (emesis) are common side effects of Dactinomycin.
- Other effects on the digestive system include diarrhea and intestinal bleeding.
- Hair loss is a frequent side effect, but usually reverses. Hair loss (called alopecia) does not threaten your health, but it can have a profound affect on how you feel about yourself.
- Many patients find the changes to their appearance, such as alopecia or changes in their fingernails, more devastating than the events that are more significant from a medical point of view.

- Other skin toxicities are seen occasionally, such as redness and increased pigment, or a severe rash.
- Radiotherapy combined with Dactinomycin can heighten the skin toxicity. It is common to have the skin in the radiation port erupt in a rash after giving Dactinomycin.

Daunorubicin

Daunorubicin is also known as rubidomycin or by its brand name Cerubidine® (Wyeth Ayerst). It is an antibiotic originally discovered in soil samples. Bacteria living in soil have evolved ways to produce many noxious compounds to help them compete with other bacteria that share their habitat. Pharmaceutical companies have been systematically collecting soil samples from around the world for years, and many of our most important antibiotics have come from different members of a bacterial family called Streptomyces.

Daunorubicin, like other anthracyclines such as Idarubicin and Doxorubicin, sticks to DNA and puts a kink in it, and that interferes with a number of the enzymes involved in maintaining the supercoil packing of DNA in chromosomes (topoisomerases).

Daunorubicin is active against several forms of leukemia.

It is given as an short intravenous infusion.

SIDE EFFECTS

- Daunorubicin causes a severe reaction to tissues it comes in contact with. Great care should be taken to make sure it all goes into the vein at the site of injection.
- Bone marrow toxicity (myelosuppression) is the most common side effect of Daunorubicin. Myelosuppression results from killing the stem cells in your bone marrow that produce new blood cells. It is detected when the cells in your blood are counted. The laboratory typically finds a reduction in white cells (neutropenia) and platelets (thrombocytopenia). The lowest counts are usually seen between day 10 and 14 after the drug was given. Your white cell counts will return to normal 10 days after this.
- Heart muscle damage (cardiotoxicity) is a major problem when using Daunorubicin. Symptoms may include fatigue, shortness of breath, especially after exercise, and an uneven heartbeat. Specific signs can be read from electrocardiograms. The more drug you have been exposed to, the greater the risk of cardiotoxicity. The damage to the heart muscle does not repair itself.
- Hair loss, including all body hair, is a frequent side effect, but usually reverses. Hair loss (called alopecia) does not threaten your health, but it can have a profound affect on how you feel about yourself.
- Many patients find the changes to their appearance, such as alopecia or changes in their fingernails, more devastating than the events that are more significant from a medical point of view.
- Rashes and other skin toxicity are rare. However, radiotherapy followed by Daunorubicin can reactivate skin toxicity from the radiation.

- Mouth sores (stomatitis) are common and unpleasant side effects. They are extremely painful, and affect your ability to swallow. It is important to keep your mouth clean and moist until this condition goes away.
- Nausea and vomiting are not as severe as with many other drugs, although there is some.
- Liver, kidney and pancreas damage has been observed in a few patients, so are possible. Daunorubicin will turn the urine red for a while. This is due to the drug being excreted and shouldn't alarm you.
- Flu-like symptoms are often reported, including fever, pain in your muscles and bone, and just feeling very sick (malaise).

Doxorubicin (Adriamycin)

Doxorubicin is also known as DOX or hydroxyl Daunorubicin or by its brand names Adriamycin® (Pharmacia and Upjohn) and Rubex® (Immunex). It is an antibiotic originally discovered in soil samples. Bacteria living in soil have evolved ways to produce many noxious compounds to help them compete with other bacteria that share their habitat. Pharmaceutical companies have been systematically collecting soil samples from around the world for years, and many of our most important antibiotics have come from different members of a bacterial family called Streptomyces.

Doxorubicin, like the other anthracyclines, such as Idarubicin and Daunorubicin, sticks to DNA and puts a kink in it, and that interferes with a number of the enzymes involved in maintaining the supercoil packing of DNA in the chromosome (topoisomerases).

Doxorubicin is active against many more kinds of tumor than its cousin Daunorubicin, and is one of the most widely used anti-cancer drugs. It is used, often in combination, to treat cancers of the lung, breast, bladder, prostate, pancreas, stomach, liver, ovary, thyroid, endometrium, sarcomas, leukemias, lymphomas, and Wilm's tumor.

Doxorubicin is usually given as an intravenous infusion over a few minutes. Sometimes very long infusions are used to control some of the side effects.

SIDE EFFECTS

- Doxorubicin causes a severe reaction to tissues it comes in contact with. Great care should be taken to make sure it all goes into the vein at the site of injection.
- Doxorubicin can also cause a reddening visible under the skin along the vein in which it is being injected. This reaction can be controlled with antihistamines and anti-inflammatories (gluco-corticoids).
- Bone marrow toxicity (myelosuppression) is the most common side effect of Doxorubicin. Myelosuppression results from killing the stem cells in your bone marrow that produce new blood cells. It is detected when the cells in your blood are counted. The laboratory typically finds a reduction in white cells (neutropenia) and platelets (thrombocytopenia). The lowest counts are usually seen between day 10 and 14 after the drug was given. Your white cell counts will return to normal 10 days after this.

- Heart muscle damage (cardiotoxicity) is a major problem when using Doxorubicin. Symptoms may include fatigue, shortness of breath, especially after exercise, and uneven heartbeat. Specific signs can be read from electrocardiograms. The more drug you have been exposed to, the greater the risk of cardiotoxicity. The damage to the heart muscle does not repair itself.
- Hair loss, involving all body hair, is a frequent side effect, but usually reverses. Hair loss (called alopecia) does not threaten your health, but it can have a profound affect on how you feel about yourself. Many patients find the changes to their appearance, such as alopecia or changes in their fingernails, more devastating than the events that are more significant from a medical point of view.
- Rashes and other skin toxicity are rare. However, if Doxorubicin is given after radiotherapy, it can reactivate skin toxicity caused by the radiation.
- Cells producing finger and toe nails are affected, and you will see increased pigment in these areas and malformation.
- Mouth sores (stomatitis) are common and unpleasant side effects. They are extremely painful, and affect your ability to swallow. It is important to keep your mouth clean and moist until this condition heals.
- Nausea and vomiting are not as severe as with many other drugs, although there is some.
- Liver, kidney and pancreas damage has been observed in a few patients, so is considered possible. Doxorubicin will turn the urine red for a while. This is due to the drug being excreted and shouldn't alarm you.
- Flu-like symptoms are often reported, including fever, pain in your muscles and bone, and just feeling very sick (malaise).
- Doxorubicin, like all the anthracyclines, may cause leukemia in some patients.
- Doxorubicin will cause urine to turn red for a while. This is due to drug being excreted and shouldn't alarm you.

Epirubicin

Epirubicin is also known as 4' epidoxorubicin or by its brand name Farmorubicin® (Pharmacia and Upjohn). It is an anthracycline, a chemically modified version of Doxorubicin, designed to improve its behavior.

Epirubicin, like its cousins Idarubicin and Doxorubicin, sticks to DNA and puts a kink in it, and that interferes with a number of the enzymes involved in maintaining the supercoil packing of DNA in the chromosome (topoisomerases).

Epirubicin is active against several tumors, including breast, stomach, ovary and lymphomas, but has not yet been approved for use by the FDA.

Epirubicin is usually given as an short intravenous infusion over a few minutes.

SIDE EFFECTS

- Epirubicin causes a severe reaction to tissues it comes in contact with. Great care should be taken to make sure it all goes into the vein at the site of injection.
- Bone marrow toxicity (myelosuppression) is the most common side effect of Epirubicin.
- Myelosuppression results from killing the stem cells in your bone marrow that produce new blood cells. It is detected when the cells in your blood are counted. The laboratory typically

finds a reduction in white cells (neutropenia) and platelets (thrombocytopenia). The lowest counts are usually seen between day 10 and 14 after the drug was given. Your white cell counts will return to normal in 21 days.

- Heart muscle damage (cardiotoxicity) is a major problem when using drugs of this type, although Epirubicin may cause less of this than its sisters. Symptoms may include fatigue, shortness of breath, especially after exercise, and uneven heartbeat. Specific signs can be read from electrocardiograms. The damage to the heart muscle does not repair itself.
- Hair loss is a frequent side effect, but usually reverses. It is less common with Epirubicin than with Doxorubicin. Hair loss (called alopecia) does not threaten your health, but it can have a profound affect on how you feel about yourself. Many patients find the changes to their appearance, such as alopecia or changes in their fingernails, more devastating than the events that are more significant from a medical point of view.
- Flu-like symptoms are reported, including fever, pain in your muscles and bone, and just feeling very sick (malaise).
- Epirubicin, like all the anthracyclines, may cause leukemia in some patients.

Etoposide (VP-16)

Etoposide, also commonly known as VP-16, or by the brand name VePesid® (Bristol-Myers Oncology) is a chemically modified version of a compound isolated from the mandrake root (also known as the May apple).

Etoposide is one of many potent drugs that have come out of folk medicine, as pharmaceutical companies isolate and study the compounds present in the plants used in old recipes. The medicinal properties of the European mandrake root is mentioned in the Bible, and is referred to in formularies throughout European history.

We believe the compound works through blocking the action of the topoisomerase enzymes. These enzymes are necessary for managing the twisting and coiling of the chromosomes that takes place when the cell is getting ready to reproduce. When VP-16 is used on cells in the laboratory, they cannot divide and the DNA is found fragmented in pieces bound with to proteins.

Etoposide is a very active compound, and is often used in combination with other drugs against certain kinds of cancer, including cancers of the lung, breast, head and neck, testis, ovaries, prostate, brain, as well as leukemia, lymphomas and sarcomas.

Etoposide is usually administered intravenously, although there are oral forms in use in some centers. Usually doctors prefer not to use the oral form because different patients absorb it differently, and it is harder to control exactly how much of it you are getting. The intravenous form is diluted to provide a long infusion time to control some of its toxicities.

SIDE EFFECTS

- Bone marrow. The primary toxicity of etoposide is that it kills the stem cells in your bone marrow that produce new blood cells. This toxicity is detected when the cells in your blood are counted. The laboratory typically finds a reduction in white cells (neutropenia) and platelets (thrombocytopenia). The lowest counts are usually 16 days after the drug was given. Bone marrow toxicity is temporary, since not all the stem cells are killed, and your white cell counts will return to normal 22 days after the drug is given.
- Nausea and vomiting (emesis) are also reported occasionally.
- Kidney or liver function is not usually a problem except in patients whose organs are impaired. These are likely to have that condition worsened by etoposide.
- Hair loss is a frequent side effect, but usually reverses. Hair loss (called alopecia) does not threaten your health, but it can have a profound affect on how you feel about yourself. Many patients find the changes to their appearance, such as alopecia or changes in their fingernails, more devastating than the events that are more significant from a medical point of view.
- Headaches and fever are common.
- Lowering of blood pressure (hypotension) is a well known problem with etoposide. The reason it is given in a slow infusion is to control the effect on blood pressure.
- Toxic effects than happen in a small proportion of patients receiving etoposide include mouth sores (mucositis), allergic reactions, damage to the heart muscle (cardiotoxicity), wheezing, and skin lesions. Less than 3% of patients become terribly tired and sleepy as a result of the drug's effect on the nervous system.
- Leukemia. As with many anti-cancer drugs, there is concern that the drugs used to treat cancer can cause a second type of cancer, like leukemia, to develop

Filgrastim (G-CSF)

Filgrastim is a genetic engineering product that is designed to mimic the natural growth control signal that triggers production of the stem cells that produce granulocytes. It also is known as Granulocyte - Colony Stimulating Factor (G-CSF), and by the brand name Neupogen® (Amgen).

G-CSF is not an anti-cancer drug, but helps manage the recovery of bone marrow after chemotherapy or radiation. Within the marrow, a series of partially differentiated stem cells are poised to replace your body's white cells depending on the needs. One type of stem cell, an intermediate in the maturation pathway, is designed to respond to a growth control signal, Filgrastim. When triggered, that cell begins to multiply and the daughters mature further, the net effect of which is to increase the number of neutrophils in the blood.

G-CSF, like PIXY-321 and GM-CSF, is used to hasten the recovery of your white blood cells. This can speed the recovery of your marrow after treatment, and it can also help you tolerate dose intensification. G-CSF is the most commonly used drug in this category, probably because many physicians believe it has fewer side effects.. The range of procedures are explained further in the section on Stem Cell Support.

It is also used in bone marrow and peripheral blood progenitor cell transplantation.

Filgrastim is given by injection, either just under the skin, or into a vein in an infusion.

SIDE EFFECTS

- The most common side effect is mild to moderate pain in your bones. This can be controlled with analgesics.

Floxuridine

Floxuridine is sold by Roche under the brand name FUDR®. It is a synthetic compound designed to mimic the natural component of DNA, thymidine, and short circuit enzymes who use it.

Floxuridine is classified as an antimetabolite, meaning it affects some of the enzymes used to synthesize or breakdown (metabolize) molecules. Antimetabolites work best on cells at a particular point (S phase) in the cell cycle, so it is most effective when the dose is given over 24 hours, to make sure all of the target cells go through S phase with the drug present.

Floxuridine is active against cancers of the colon, prostate, mouth, pancreas, liver and biliary tract, ovaries, and kidney.

Floxuridine is administered by injection directly into an artery in the organ containing the tumor.

SIDE EFFECTS

- Many of the side effects reported for Floxuridine have to do with the problems of intra-arterial injection. Leakage at the site, damage to the artery, blocked catheters are all problems.
- Bone marrow toxicity (myelosuppression) is the most common side effect of Floxuridine.
- This is a side effect of killing the stem cells in your bone marrow that produce new blood cells. It is detected when the cells in your blood are counted. The laboratory typically finds a reduction in white cells (neutropenia) and platelet reduction (thrombocytopenia).
- Nausea and vomiting (emesis) are common side effects of Floxuridine. Even with combinations of corticosteroids and new anti-emetic drugs, many patients still have terrible nausea.
- Other effects on the digestive system include abdominal cramps, pain, severe diarrhea and intestinal bleeding.
- Mouth sores (mucositis) are common and very unpleasant side effects. They are extremely painful, and affect your ability to swallow. It is important to keep your mouth clean and moist until this condition goes away.
- Skin toxicities include rash and effects on your nail formation.
- Hair loss is a frequent side effect, but usually reverses. Hair loss (called alopecia) does not threaten your health, but it can have a profound affect on how you feel about yourself.

- Many patients find the changes to their appearance, such as alopecia or changes in their fingernails, more devastating than the events that are more significant from a medical point of view.

Fludarabine

Fludarabine is also known as 2-fluoro-Ara-AMP, FLAMP or by the brand name Fludara® (Berlex). It is a new synthetic compound designed to mimic the natural component of DNA, adenine, and short circuit enzymes who use it.

Fludarabine is classified as an antimetabolite, meaning it affects some of the enzymes used to synthesize or breakdown (metabolize) molecules. Antimetabolites work best on cells at a particular point (S phase) in the cell cycle, so it is most effective when the dose is given over 24 hours, to make sure all of the target cells go through S phase with the drug present.

Fludarabine is active against some forms of leukemia, and lymphoma.

Fludarabine is administered intravenously in a long infusion. Sometimes it is given in a series of daily short infusions.

SIDE EFFECTS

- Bone marrow toxicity (myelosuppression) is the most common side effect of Fludarabine. Myelosuppression results from killing the stem cells in your bone marrow that produce new blood cells. It is detected when the cells in your blood are counted. The laboratory typically finds a reduction in white cells (neutropenia) and platelet reduction (thrombocytopenia).
- Nausea and vomiting (emesis) are common side effects of Fludarabine. Even with combinations of corticosteroids and anti-emetic drugs, many patients still have terrible nausea.
- Other effects on the digestive system include abdominal cramps, pain, severe diarrhea and intestinal bleeding.
- Central nervous system toxicity can be severe at high doses. This can include blindness, seizures and even coma.
- Skin toxicities include rash and effects on your nails formation.
- Hair loss is a frequent side effect, but usually reverses. Hair loss (called alopecia) does not threaten your health, but it can have a profound affect on how you feel about yourself. Many patients find the changes to their appearance, such as alopecia or changes in their fingernails, more devastating than the events that are more significant from a medical point of view.

5-Fluorouracil (5FU)

5- Fluorouracil, or 5-FU is sold by Roche under the brand name Fluorouracil. It is a synthetic compound designed to mimic the natural component of DNA, thymidine, and short circuit enzymes who use it. It is the most widely used antimetabolite because of the range of tumors against which it is active.

5- Fluorouracil is classified as an antimetabolite, meaning it affects some of the enzymes used to synthesize or breakdown (metabolize) molecules. Antimetabolites work best on cells at a particular point (S phase) in the <u>cell cycle</u>, so it is most effective when the dose is given over 24 hours, to make sure all of the target cells go through S phase in the presence of the drug.

5- Fluorouracil is one of the few drugs that are active against colon cancer, and is used to treat a variety of solid tumors, often in combination with other agents. These include cancers of the liver, head and neck, kidney, stomach, pancreas, lung and breast. There has been a revival of interest using 5-Fluorouracil in treatment combinations since the finding that Leucovorin helps control some of the toxicities.

5- Fluorouracil is administered by injection into your veins either quickly or over a long infusion (over 1 to 4 days).

SIDE EFFECTS

- Bone marrow toxicity (myelosuppression) is the most common side effect of 5- Fluorouracil. This kind of toxicity results from killing the stem cells in your bone marrow that produce new blood cells. It is detected when the cells in your blood are counted. The laboratory typically finds a reduction in white cells (neutropenia) and platelets (thrombocytopenia). Cell counts reach the lowest levels between day 7 and 14.
- Mouth sores (stomatitis) are common and very unpleasant side effects of 5-Fluorouracil. These may not appear for 5 to 8 days. They are extremely painful, and affect your ability to swallow. Some patients have such a severe problem that dosing has to be discontinued. It is important to keep your mouth clean and moist until this condition goes away.
- Nausea and vomiting (emesis) are also common side effects of 5- Fluorouracil. Even with combinations of corticosteroids and new anti-emetic drugs, many patients still have terrible nausea.
- Other effects on the digestive system include inflammation of the esophagus, pain, severe diarrhea, ulcers and intestinal bleeding.
- Skin toxicities include rash and effects on finger and toe nail formation. It is not uncommon to develop a rash, which will go away soon. The rash may be sensitive to sunlight.
- Darkening of the skin around the veins in which the 5-Fluorouracil is infused is often observed. You may experience darkening of the skin at the base of your nails or face and hands.
- The palms and soles of the feet may become reddish and lose sensitivity to touch.
- Hair loss is a frequent side effect, but usually reverses. Hair loss (called alopecia) does not threaten your health, but it can have a profound affect on how you feel about yourself. Many patients find the changes to their appearance, such as alopecia or changes in their fingernails, more devastating than the events that are more significant from a medical point of view.
- Damage to the central nervous system is rare, but has been reported. Symptoms include headache, problems seeing or lack of coordination.
- Heart muscle damage, including cardiac arrest, has been reported in a small number of patients.

Fluoxymesterone

Fluoxymesterone, also known as Halotestin® (Pharmacia and Upjohn) is a synthetic compound designed to mimic the male steroid hormone androgen. It is not an anti-cancer drug, but is used as hormone therapy to control breast cancer growth, similar to Tamoxifen.

Estrogen, like many signal hormones, is produced at one site (the ovaries) whence it circulates to the organs that need to respond to the signal. Among the many estrogen responsive cells are those in the breasts, which prepare for the potential pregnancy during the menstrual cycle. This response by the cells occurs because there is an estrogen receptor on them, to which estrogen binds, which event then triggers a series of changes in cell activity.

The daughters of the cell that initiated the tumor in breast cancer will have estrogen receptors in about two thirds of patients. Years ago it was common to remove the ovaries from women with breast cancer, because the cancer cells stopped growing when the estrogen was removed. Now we duplicate this effect by treating with drugs which tie up the estrogen receptors so they can't respond to estrogen.

Fluoxymesterone is given orally as a tablet.

SIDE EFFECTS

- Virilization is sometimes observed. This might include changes in menstrual cycle, increased facial hair, deepening of the voice, or acne. Clitoral enlargement is another aspect of the spectrum of virilization responses.
- Fluid retention, symptomatic of changes in electrolytes are another well known side effect of Fluoxymesterone. This group of side effects include possible kidney or liver damage, and hypercalcemia.

Furosemide

Furosemide, or Lasix® (Hoechst-Roussel) is not an anti-cancer drug, but a drug used to help manage the side effects of certain cancer drugs. It works by blocking the uptake of salts in the kidney. This changes the osmotic balance in the critical and tightly regulated flow of fluids out of the blood in the kidney.

Furosemide increases the amount of water that is passed into the bladder and excreted as urine. It is used to reduce water retention, which alleviates the edema that results from extensive removal of lymph nodes.

Furosemide is also used to increase the flow of fluid through the kidney to wash out those drugs that cause nephrotoxicity and reduce the potential for damage.

Furosemide is usually given orally, as a tablet, but injectable solutions are also available.

- Furosemide is well tolerated, however, in patients with kidney problems or who are taking medication that could affect the kidney careful monitoring is required.
- Dehydration is potentially a problem; enough fluids are required, such as i.v. solutions, to balance those excreted.
- Damage to the ear.

Gallium nitrate

Gallium nitrate may be known by the brand name Ganite® (Fujisawa). It is not an anti-cancer agent but is used to treat one of the side effects of cancer (hypercalcemia).

Gallium nitrate inhibits bone absorption by complexing with the calcium being laid down by osteoblasts. The complexed crystal is not as easily absorbed by osteoclasts, which effectively lowers the amount of calcium circulating in the blood and restoring the calcium levels to normal range.

Gallium nitrate is given by intravenous infusion over 24 hr.

- At the dose levels used to treat hypercalcemia there are few side effects with Gallium nitrate. The effects are: too little calcium (hypocalcemia), decreased levels of other electrolytes, such as bicarbonate, and lowering of blood pressure.

Gemcitabine

Gemcitabine is an experimental new drug that is currently being investigated in clinical trials. It is a synthetic compound designed to imitate the natural constituent of DNA, cytosine, similar to Cytarabine.

Gemcitabine is classified as an antimetabolite, meaning it affects some of the enzymes used to synthesize or breakdown (metabolize) molecules.

Gemcitabine must be activated by the cell in order to be effective, and the rate of conversion affects its effectiveness and its toxicity.

Gemcitabine is administered either as an intravenous infusion or by injection just below the skin (subcutaneous) or into the muscle (intramuscular).

- Bone marrow toxicity (myelosuppression) is the most common side effect of Gemcitabine. This is a side effect of killing the stem cells in your bone marrow that produce new blood cells. It is detected when the cells in your blood are counted. The laboratory typically finds a reduction in platelets (thrombocytopenia), with less effect on neutrophils.

- Flushing of the skin, usually with rashes on the palms, soles of the feet, chest and neck are reported.
- Fever like symptoms are often reported, including pain in your muscles and bone, and just feeling very sick (malaise).

Idarubicin

Idarubicin's brand name is Idamycin® (Pharmacia and Upjohn). It is a chemically altered form of doxorubicin, designed to be more effective and less toxic.

Idarubicin, like other anthracyclines, sticks to DNA and puts a kink in it, and that interferes with a number of the enzymes involved in maintaining the supercoil packing of DNA in the cell (topoisomerases).

Idarubicin is active against many types of leukemia and lymphomas.

Idarubicin is usually given as an intravenous infusion over a few minutes.

SIDE EFFECTS

- Idarubicin causes a severe reaction to tissues it comes in contact with. Great care should be taken to make sure it all goes into the vein at the site of injection.
- Idarubicin can also cause a reddening visible under the skin along the vein in which it is being injected. This reaction can be controlled with antihistamines and anti-inflammatories (gluco-corticoids).
- Bone marrow toxicity (myelosuppression) is the most common side effect of Idarubicin. This is a side effect of killing the stem cells in your bone marrow that produce new blood cells. It is detected when the cells in your blood are counted. The laboratory typically finds a reduction in white cells (neutropenia) and platelets (thrombocytopenia). The lowest counts are usually seen around day 10 after the drug was given. Your white cell counts will return to normal 5 to 10 days after this.
- Heart muscle damage (cardiotoxicity) is a problem when using Idarubicin, although it may be less severe than with doxorubicin. Symptoms may include fatigue, shortness of breath, especially after exercise, and uneven heartbeat. Specific signs can be read from electrocardiograms. The more drug you have been exposed to, the greater the risk of cardiotoxicity. The damage to the heart muscle does not repair itself.
- Nausea and vomiting (emesis) are experienced by most patients about 30 minutes after the dose, and can be severe. They can be controlled with drugs designed for that purpose.
- Mouth sores (stomatitis) are common and unpleasant side effects. They are extremely painful, and affect your ability to swallow. It is important to keep your mouth clean and moist until this condition goes away.
- Diarrhea is also common.
- Hair loss, including all body hair, is a frequent side effect, but usually reverses. Hair loss (called alopecia) does not threaten your health, but it can have a profound affect on how you feel about yourself. Many patients find the changes to their appearance, such as alopecia or changes in their fingernails, more devastating than the events that are more significant from a medical point of view.

- Liver, kidney and pancreas damage has been observed in many patients. These may not have symptoms, but will show up when your blood is analyzed.
- Idarubicin will turn the urine red for a while. This is due to the drug being excreted and shouldn't alarm you.
- Flu-like symptoms are often reported, including fever, pain in your muscles and bone, and just feeling very sick (malaise).
- Idarubicin, like all the anthracyclines, may cause leukemia in some patients.

Ifosfamide

Ifosfamide is also known as isophosphamide or by the brand names IFEX® (Bristol Myers Oncology) or Holoxan® (Astra). It is a synthetic member of the nitrogen mustard family, which includes Chlorambucil and Cyclophosphamide. These compounds were originally exploited for chemical warfare during World War I. The first drugs used in anti-cancer chemotherapy were nitrogen mustards.

All the nitrogen mustard drugs convert to an active species once they get inside a cell. Once converted, they are highly interactive with a number of different molecules, but the most important target is the cell's DNA. They bind to DNA and crosslink the strands (called alkylation), which prevents DNA from being duplicated, and either kills the cell or stops it from dividing. The various nitrogen mustards differ in potency, toxicity and what kind of tumors they are active against. The differences are attributed to the rate they get into various cells, the rate they convert, and what kind of damage they inflict once there.

Ifosfamide is effective against may types of cancer, including cancers of the lung, ovary, testis, breast. leukemias sarcomas and lymphomas. It is often a component of mixed drug chemotherapy (see the table at the beginning of this section).

Ifosfamide can be given by intravenous infusion over 30 minutes or in a long infusion over 5 days.

SIDE EFFECTS

- Bladder damage is the most severe side effect of Ifosfamide, no matter the rate of infusion. Frequently blood is observed in the urine which leads to cystitis. You will be hydrated, or given lots of fluids to increase the flow rate through the kidneys and bladder to control this condition. Mesna is a drug that is frequently given along with Ifosfamide to help control bladder damage.
- Kidney damage (nephrotoxicity) often is seen, which is detected in the chemical tests of your blood
- Gastrointestinal toxicity, including anorexia, nausea and vomiting is common. Nausea usually starts a few hours after the dose, and will persist for about 3 days.
- Bone marrow toxicity (myelosuppression) is another side effect of Ifosfamide, but is not severe.

- This is a side effect of killing the stem cells in your bone marrow that produce new blood cells. This toxicity is detected when the cells in your blood are counted. The laboratory typically finds a reduction in white cells (neutropenia).
- Nerve damage, which usually (but doesn't always) go away, is known to happen, especially with large doses. This is detected as sleepiness or confusion, and sometimes seizures.
- Hair loss is a frequent side effect, but usually reverses. Hair loss (called alopecia) does not threaten your health, but it can have a profound affect on how you feel about yourself. Many patients find the changes to their appearance, such as alopecia or changes in their fingernails, more devastating than the events that are more significant from a medical point of view.

Interferon Alpha

Interferon Alpha is a drug that imitates one of the natural components of your immune system. It is one of the tools in the <u>Biological Therapy</u> category. Interferons were discovered as part of the armament your immune system cells produce to fight viruses and cancer. Recently we have discovered techniques for making human gene products by tricking bacteria to produce them by fermentation. Several Interferon Alpha products are available, including Intron® A (Schering), Roferon® A (Roche), Alferon® N (Purdue Frederick) and Wellferon® (Glaxo Wellcome). They all differ in detail, but are treated together here for simplicity.

Interferon Alpha is a natural human protein produced by white blood cells. They bind to cells that have an Interferon receptor on their surface and trigger the cell to turn on a number of genes which ultimately fight viral infections. While we do not fully understand the cascade of effects, we know that multiple components of the immune system become mobilized, and there is an anti-tumor effect.

Interferon Alpha is approved for use against Hairy Cell Leukemia and AIDS-associated Kaposi's Sarcoma. It is also being studied as part of combination therapies in a number of other types of cancer, including kidney, melanoma, myeloma and Kaposi's sarcoma.

Interferon Alpha is given by injection, either just below the skin or into the muscle.

SIDE EFFECTS

- The major side effect are flu-like symptoms, such as fever, chills, muscle pain, headaches and an overall miserable feeling (malaise).
- An extension of these effects is fatigue, which may be so intense as to stop dosing.
- Weight loss and nausea may happen at high doses.
- Some patients have mild toxicity to their bone marrow, or liver.

Interleukins

Interleukins are proteins produced by white blood cells as part of their armory to fight infections and other diseases. There are at least 15 Interleukins, and more will likely be discovered as we probe the workings of the immune system. Some are experimental agents being studied in different settings as we try to understand how to use the agents of Biological Therapy.

Interleukin-1 (IL-1) actually consists of two types, alpha and beta. They are produced by the cells known as monocytes, and have a powerful effect on several systems in fighting disease. IL-1 acts directly to stimulate stem cells in the bone marrow to mobilize, and it induces the production of a number of growth factors that further stimulate the production of new white blood cells. IL-1 acts directly on the brain to produce fever, which is a serious limitation in using this compound. Il-1 activates the cell killing activity of some T-lymphocytes, and it activates neutrophils. It is part of a complex signaling system, and triggers the release of a number of other interleukins and factors.

Interleukin-2 or Aldesleukin, is produced by mature T lymphocytes. IL-2 was originally discovered as a factor that induces T lymphocytes to multiply. It has no anti-tumor activity by itself, but activates certain lymphocytes to become potent tumor cell killers. In clinical trials IL-2 has had some stunning successes, but not frequently enough. We are actively trying to find ways to combine this with other compounds to increase the frequency of these responses.

Interleukin-3 is a growth factor and stimulates the production of a wide range of blood cells in the marrow, including red cells, platelets as well as monocytes and granulocytes. IL-3 is normally produced as a signal molecule from activated T lymphocytes. It does not have direct anti-tumor activity, but it is being studied as an important link in the complex system our bodies mount to fight disease.

Interleukin-11 is an experimental drug that is being tested as a growth factor to stimulate production of platelets. We have growth factors to hasten the replacement of neutorphils, but not for platelets. Interleukin-11 is one of the promising candidates for managing this side effect.

Leucovorin

Leucovorin is a synthetic compound designed to mimic the natural vitamin, folic acid, and disrupt cell enzymes that use it. It is not an anti-cancer agent, but a drug used to modify the effects of other drugs which depend on folic acid for their activity. It is also known as folinic acid, citrovorum factor, or by the brand name Wellcovorin® (Burroughs Wellcome).

Leucovorin was originally used to "rescue" patients being treated with Methotrexate. Methotrexate is a potent blocker of enzymes that use the folic acid vitamin, and Leucovorin was used to rescue patients who were in trouble because they couldn't handle the methotrexate. More recently, Leucovorin has been shown useful in making 5-Fluorouracil more active and less toxic as well.

Leucovorin is administered orally as a tablet or intravenously.

SIDE EFFECTS

- The only side effects are rare cases of allergic reactions.

Leuprolide

Leuprolide (brand name Lupron®) is a synthetic compound designed to mimic the natural peptide hormone LH-RH. It is not an anti-cancer agent, but is used in the treatment of prostate cancer to shut off production of Testosterone.

Leutinizing Hormone Releasing Hormone, or LH-RH, is also known as Gonadotropin-Releasing Hormone. The natural hormone acts on the pituitary gland to stimulate production of signals that induce the testes to produce Testosterone. Prostate cancer cells are stimulated by Testosterone, and lowering the levels of this hormone helps control their growth.

Leuprolide is administered as an injection, either under the skin or into the muscle.

SIDE EFFECTS

- Hot flashes, ranging in intensity from mild to intense.

Liposomes

Liposomes are not, by themselves, drugs. They are tiny artificial cells that are filled with drugs, such as those used to treat cancer. Liposomes are used to alter the way anti-cancer drugs interact with the body. While no liposomal forms of drugs are currently approved by the FDA, several are in advanced stages of testing. We don't know enough about them to judge how safe and effective they are or how they compare to each other.

Liposomal cells are made of the same material that the outer membrane of real cells is built from. As they enter the bloodstream, they circulate as cells, protecting many tissues from the side effects of the drug they contain. Liposomes eventually collect in certain tissues, depending on their construction, and release their contents, much like the Trojan horse of legend.

Anti-cancer drugs delivered in liposomes include Doxorubicin, Daunorubicin, Tretinoin, and Cytarabine, and other agents are near testing. The clinical trials of these drugs seem to indicate that the liposome form of the drug has less toxicity than pure drug. This may be especially important for the anthracycline drugs, if the cardiotoxicity can be reduced or eliminated (Cardiotoxicity, unlike myelosuppression, is irreversible).

Liposome drugs are administered by injection into a vein, over several minutes.

SIDE EFFECTS

- Myelosuppression is the dose limiting toxicity for most liposome drugs, because the bone marrow is a major site where liposomes accumulate.
- Other toxicities will be revealed as the clinical trials progress.

Lomustine (CCNU)

Lomustine is also known as CCNU, and by its brand name of CeeNU® (Bristol Myers Oncology). It is a synthetic nitrosourea compound, designed to be more potent and less toxic than Carmustine.

It is an alkylating agent, and converts to a short lived, highly reactive molecule, which is the form that actually causes the damage. Once the molecule is armed, it binds to DNA and proteins, which stops them from being effective and blocks the cell from duplicating. It has been used against many types of cancer, including cancers of the brain, kidney and lung, lymphomas and melanoma.

Lomustine is given orally, as a capsule.

SIDE EFFECTS

- Toxicity to the Bone marrow (myelosuppression) is the most significant side effect with Lomustine. Depletion of the marrow takes longer than with most anti-cancer drugs, but is severe.
- Myelosuppression is caused by killing the stem cells in your bone marrow that produce new blood cells. It is detected when the cells in your blood are counted. The laboratory typically finds a reduction in white cells (leukopenia) and platelets (thrombocytopenia). The lowest white cell and platelet counts are usually seen 3 to 5 weeks after the drug is given. Bone marrow toxicity is temporary, since not all the stem cells are killed, and your white cell counts will return to normal 4 to 8 weeks after the drug is given. If your marrow has already been depleted by previous treatments, this toxicity can be even more severe.
- Nausea and vomiting (emesis) are very common side effects, and start 2 to 6 hours after taking the drug. Diarrhea is less common and is not severe.
- Mouth sores (stomatitis), and hair loss are reported.
- Kidney damage is sometimes seen with Lomustine therapy. These show up in test results when your blood is analyzed, and usually go away without problems, but very high doses may cause kidney failure.
- A small number of patients suffer neurologic toxicity, which is detected as confusion or lack of coordination.

Mechlorethamine

Mechlorethamine, or nitrogen mustard (brand name Mustargen®, Merck) was produced during the first World War as a variant of mustard gas. It was one of the first chemical agents used to treat cancer in the 1940s.

The demonstration that a combination of agents known as MOPP in 1970 resulted in a high cure rate for Hodgkin's Lymphoma was a watershed in treatment of cancer with chemical therapies. Mechlorethamine is the "M" in MOPP. It is also used to treat non-Hodgkin's lymphoma, cancer of the lung and others.

All the nitrogen mustard drugs convert to an active species once they get inside a cell. Once converted, they are highly interactive with a number of different molecules, but the most important target is the cell's DNA. They bind to DNA and crosslink the strands (called alkylation), which prevents DNA from being duplicated, and either kills the cell or stops it from dividing. The various nitrogen mustards differ in potency, toxicity and what kind of tumors they are active against. The differences are attributed to the rate they get into various cells, the rate they convert, and what kind of damage they inflict once there.

Mechlorethamine is administered by injection into a vein.

SIDE EFFECTS

- Great care should be taken that Mechlorethamine not contact the skin during injection. Contact on the skin will cause a chemical burn which can be quite nasty.
- Sometimes the vein itself becomes inflamed, which can be so severe treatment has to be stopped.
- Bone marrow toxicity (myelosuppression) is the most common side effect of Mechlorethamine. This is a side effect of killing the stem cells in your bone marrow that produce new blood cells. It is detected when the cells in your blood are counted. The laboratory typically finds a reduction in white cells (neutropenia). The lowest counts are usually seen between day 8 and 14 after the drug was given. Your white cell counts will return to normal 10 to 20 days after this. Platelet reduction (thrombocytopenia) can sometimes be severe, causing bleeding.
- Nausea and vomiting (emesis) are common side effects of Mechlorethamine. It usually starts within 3 hours, and diminishes after 8 hours. Even with combinations of corticosteroids and anti-emetic drugs, many patients still have terrible nausea.
- Other effects on the digestive system include diarrhea and intestinal bleeding.
- Skin rashes occur infrequently.
- Affects on sperm production or irregular menstrual cycle should be anticipated.
- Neurological problems, such as ringing in your ears, weakness, drowsiness or headaches are infrequent but can happen.

Melphalan

Melphalan is another member of the nitrogen mustard family of alkylating agents, like Cyclophosphamide, Ifosfamide, Mechlorethamine and Busulfan. It is some-times known as PAM, Phenylalanine Mustard, L-Sarcolysine or by the brand name Alkeran® (Glaxo-Wellcome).

The nitrogen mustard family of agents are descendants of the mustard gas used in chemical warfare during World War I. They were the first drugs used to selectively kill tumor cells during the 1940s.

All the nitrogen mustard drugs convert to an active species once they get inside a cell. Once converted, they are highly interactive with a number of different molecules, but the most important target is the cell's DNA. They bind to DNA and crosslink the strands (called alkylation), which prevents DNA from being duplicated, and either kills the cell or stops it from dividing. The various nitrogen mustards differ in potency, toxicity and what kind of tumors they are active against. The differences are attributed to the rate they get into various cells, the rate they convert, and what kind of damage they inflict once there.

Melphalan is active against a number of different tumors, including myeloma, ovarian, testicular and breast cancer.

Melphalan is given either orally, as a tablet, or into the vein by slow infusion over thirty minutes.

SIDE EFFECTS

- Bone marrow toxicity (myelosuppression) is the most common side effect of Melphelan. This is a side effect of killing the stem cells in your bone marrow that produce new blood cells. It is detected when the cells in your blood are counted. The laboratory typically finds a reduction in white cells (neutropenia). The lowest counts are usually seen about 14 days after the drug was given, but may decline further due to cumulative effects. Platelet reduction (thrombo-cytopenia) is most severe by day 21.
- There is some evidence that prolonged exposure to Melphalan can increase the risk of developing some form of leukemia later on.
- Hair loss (alopecia) does not happen to most patients taking Melphalan, but does for some. Your hair will grow back, but it can be disturbing.
- Nausea and vomiting (emesis) are common side effects for patients taking the oral form, but not the intravenous.
- Other effects on the digestive system include mouth sores, diarrhea and intestinal bleeding. Occasionally, patients who take Melphalan develop lung damage. These are usually patients who have been taking the oral form for a long term.

6-Mercaptopurine

6-Mercaptopurine, or Purinethol® (Glaxo-Wellcome) is a small synthetic molecule designed to imitate the natural product, hypoxanthine, which is used to make some components of DNA.

It is classified as an antimetabolite, similar to Thioguanine, or Pentostatin. It must be activated inside the cell by fooling some of the enzymes used to produce DNA. It interferes with several biochemical pathways to kill the cell, including DNA and RNA synthesis.

It is active against several forms of leukemia.

6-Mercaptopurine is given orally as a tablet.

SIDE EFFECTS

- Bone marrow toxicity (myelosuppression) is the most common side effect of 6-Mercaptopurine, but is not severe at the normal doses. This is a side effect of killing the stem cells in your bone marrow that produce new blood cells. It is detected when the cells in your blood are counted. The laboratory typically finds a reduction in white cells (neutropenia) and platelets (thrombocytopenia). The lowest counts are usually seen between day 11 and 23 after the drug was given. Your white cell counts will return to normal 10 days after this.
- Hair loss is a frequent side effect, but usually reverses. Hair loss (called alopecia) does not threaten your health, but it can have a profound affect on how you feel about yourself. Many patients find the changes to their appearance, such as alopecia or changes in their fingernails, more devastating than the events that are more significant from a medical point of view.
- Nausea and vomiting (emesis) are only occasionally side effects of 6-Mercaptopurine.
- Other rare effects on the digestive system include diarrhea and intestinal bleeding.
- Mouth sores (stomatitis) are common and very unpleasant side effects. They are extremely painful, and affect your ability to swallow. It is important to keep your mouth clean and moist until this condition goes away.
- Liver damage has been observed in a few patients, so is considered possible. It can be severe in a few instances.
- Blood in the urine is sometimes seen with high doses.
- Flushing of the skin, and sometimes rashes are reported.
- Flu-like symptoms are often reported, including fever, pain in your muscles and bone, and just feeling very sick (malaise).

Mesna

Mesna is a small synthetic compound that is used to reduce the effects of certain anti-cancer drugs on the kidneys. It is known by a number of different brand names, including Uromitexan® (Astra-Werke), Mesnex® (Bristol-Myers Oncology) and Mistabron® (UCB).

Certain alkylating agents, like Cyclophosphamide and Ifosfamide, cause the formation of poisonous compounds (such as acrolein) in your kidneys. Mesna binds to these and neutralizes them before they cause too much damage. Neutralizing these toxins has nothing to do with the anti-cancer effects of these drugs, but controlling the toxins enables you to receive enough of these drugs to control your disease.

Mesna is administered either orally as a liquid or into the vein.

SIDE EFFECTS

- At the doses usually given there are few side effects from Mesna. The oral form has an unpleasant taste. Nausea, and mild diarrhea are occasionally experienced.

Methotrexate

Methotrexate is known by a number of different names, including amthopterin, MTX, and the brand names Folex®. Mexate® and Rheumatrex®. Methotrexate was one of the first compounds specifically designed to block a key enzyme that produces the building blocks of DNA and RNA.

Methotrexate is an antimetabolite, and is only effective during one sector of the cell cycle, S phase. It mimics the enzyme cofactor folic acid, preventing the enzyme that uses that cofactor from working. As a result the cell cannot make new DNA or RNA.

Methotrexate can be given in doses that would be fatal, were it not possible to "rescue" you with the related compound, Leucovorin, which neutralizes the toxicity quickly. This combination is used as a way of overcoming some resistant cells.

Methotrexate is active against a number of different types of cancer, including lung cancer, head and neck cancer, sarcoma, leukemia, tumors of the breast, lung, stomach, esophagus, testis and lymphomas. It is often used as part of a mixture of agents. It is one of the few anti-cancer drugs that is also used for other diseases, including psoriasis and rheumatoid arthritis.

Methotrexate is given either orally, as a tablet, or by injection into either a muscle or as an intravenous infusion.

SIDE EFFECTS

- Bone marrow toxicity (myelosuppression) is the most common side effect of Methotrexate. This is a side effect of killing the stem cells in your bone marrow that produce new blood cells. It is detected when the cells in your blood are counted. First, there is a reduction in your red blood cells (anemia), followed by a reduction in white cells (neutropenia). The lowest counts are usually seen between day 4 and 7 after the drug was given, which may occasionally be followed by an additional depression in cell numbers around day 21. Platelet reduction (thrombocytopenia) is most severe between 5 and 12 days.

- Nausea and vomiting (emesis) are common side effects of Methotrexate. Other effects on the digestive system include diarrhea and intestinal bleeding. Sometimes the lining of the digestive track gets severely irritated, and it may perforate, with disastrous consequences.
- Mouth sores (stomatitis) are common and very unpleasant side effects, and can be severe. They are extremely painful, and affect your ability to swallow. You may have to interrupt treatment if the mouth sores erupt into ulcers in the mouth or stomach. It is important to keep your mouth clean and moist until this condition goes away.
- Hair loss is a frequent side effect, but usually reverses. Hair loss (called alopecia) does not threaten your health, but it can have a profound affect on how you feel about yourself. Many patients find the changes to their appearance, such as alopecia or changes in their fingernails, more devastating than the events that are more significant from a medical point of view.
- Liver damage has been observed in some patients, especially at high doses. This will cause certain blood chemistry tests to show elevated enzyme levels, and increased bilirubin. Usually these return to normal within a week or so, but occasionally persistent liver damage happens.
- Flushing of the skin, an itching or burning sensation, and rashes are common.
- Nerve damage, which usually goes away, is known to happen, especially with large doses. This is detected as dizziness or blurred vision.

Mitomycin-C

Mitomycin-C, whose brand name is Mutamycin® (Bristol-Myers Oncology), is an antibiotic originally discovered in soil samples. Bacteria living in soil have evolved ways to produce many noxious compounds to help them compete with other bacteria that share their habitat. Pharmaceutical companies have been systematically collecting soil samples from around the world for years, and many of our most important antibiotics have come from different members of this bacterial family called Streptomyces.

Mitomycin-C is an alkylating agent that becomes activated once it gets inside the cell. Once armed, it binds (alkylates) cell DNA and proteins, causing cross-linking and strand breaks. The effect is to prevent the cell from replicating its DNA.

Mitomycin-C is active against a number of different tumor types, including cancer of the stomach, colon, anus, pancreas, cervix, breast and lung cancer.

Mitomycin-C is given by injection into the vein, usually by an infusion over many hours.

SIDE EFFECTS

- Mitomycin-C causes a severe reaction to tissues it comes in contact with. Great care should be taken to make sure it all goes into the vein at the site of injection.
- Bone marrow toxicity (myelosuppression) is the most common side effect of Mitomycin-C. Like the nitosoureas, Mitomycin-C affects on the bone marrow can be cumulative and slow recovering. This is a side effect of killing the stem cells in your bone marrow that produce new blood cells. It is detected when the cells in your blood are counted. The laboratory typically

finds a reduction in red cells (anemia), white cells (neutropenia) or platelets (thrombocytopenia).

- Hair loss is a frequent side effect, but usually reverses. Hair loss (called alopecia) does not threaten your health, but it can have a profound affect on how you feel about yourself. Many patients find the changes to their appearance, such as alopecia or changes in their fingernails, more devastating than the events that are more significant from a medical point of view.
- Nausea and vomiting (emesis) often follow Mitomycin-C dosing, but are not severe.
- Other effects on the digestive system include diarrhea and intestinal bleeding.
- Mouth sores (stomatitis) may erupt but are not as severe as with other anti-cancer drugs. They are extremely painful, and affect your ability to swallow. It is important to keep your mouth clean and moist until this condition goes away.
- Kidney damage (nephrotoxicity) may be observed in the blood chemistry tests, but is usually not severe and resolves itself.
- At high doses, some patients develop a blood disease called microangiopathic hemolytic anemia, which can be fatal because of its effects on the kidneys. MAHA may not develop for weeks after the last dose was administered.
- Flushing of the skin, and sometimes rashes on the palms, soles of the feet, chest and neck are reported.
- Flu-like symptoms are often reported, including fever, pain in your muscles and bone, and just feeling very sick (malaise).

Mitoxantrone

Mitoxantrone is also known by the brand name Novantrone® (Immunex). It is a synthetic compound similar in structure and properties to the anthracyclines, a class of antibiotics that includes Doxorubicin and Idarubicin.

Like the anthracyclines, Mitoxantrone interacts with DNA and we believe that interaction affects the ability of the topoisomerase enzymes to cope with the relaxation of the supercoils during replication, and causes breaks in the DNA.

Mitoxantrone is active against a number of different types of cancer, including leukemia, carcinomas of the breast and ovaries.

Mitoxantrone is given into the vein usually by slow infusion over thirty minutes.

SIDE EFFECTS

- Bone marrow toxicity (myelosuppression) is the most common side effect of Mitoxantrone. This is a side effect of killing the stem cells in your bone marrow that produce new blood cells. It is detected when the cells in your blood are counted. The laboratory typically finds a reduction in white cells (neutropenia). The lowest counts are usually seen between day 10 and 4 after the drug was given. Your white cell counts will return to normal 10 days after this.
- Nausea and vomiting (emesis) are common side effects of Mitoxantrone, but are not severe. Even with combinations of corticosteroids and these new drugs, many patients still have terrible nausea.

- Mouth sores (stomatitis) are common and very unpleasant side effects. They can be painful, and affect your ability to swallow. It is important to keep your mouth clean and moist until this condition goes away.
- Hair loss (alopecia) is not as common as with most anti-cancer drugs, but is experienced sometimes. Your hair will grow back, but it is disturbing to some.
- Toxicity to the heart muscle (cardiotoxicity) is an irreversible side effect that limits the amount of drug you can receive. This is a potentially fatal consequence of receiving too much drug, and must be monitored carefully.

Octreotide

Octreotide, or Sandostatin® (Novartis) is a synthetic peptide designed to mimic the natural peptide hormone, Somatostatin.

Somatostatin is produced by the hypothalamus in the brain, and is one of the molecular thermostats that regulates the level of activity of a number of interrelated activities. Octreotide substitutes for that activity in patients whose cancer causes a derangement of the normal control mechanisms. It is not an anti-tumor agent, but helps manage some of the symptoms in patients with cancer of pancreatic cells that produce vasoactive intestinal peptides, as well as other endocrine system tumors.

Octreotide is administered as an injection just below the skin.

SIDE EFFECTS

- Irritation of the digestive system may cause nausea, stomach cramps of diarrhea in a few patients.
- Other, rare effects are dizziness, changes in blood pressure (either up or down), anxiety, changes in blood sugar levels (either up or down), and skin flushing.

Ondansetron

Ondansetron, or Zofran® (Glaxo Wellcome) is not an anti-cancer drug, but is an anti-emetic. It is used to control the nausea and vomiting (emesis) that often result when certain anti-cancer drugs are used. Ondansetron blocks those signals from the intestine that trigger the complex series of events that leads to emesis.

Ondansetron is given by injection, into a vein.

SIDE EFFECTS

- Constipation is a frequent side effect. Some patients experience a rash, and there is some evidence of liver toxicity, probably in patients whose liver is not working well to begin with.

Paclitaxel (Taxol)

Paclitaxel, or Taxol® (Bristol-Myers Oncology) is a natural compound that is purified from the bark and needles of the western yew tree. It has a complex structure that has so far defied efforts to produce it by chemical synthesis. It was discovered over twenty years ago, but only recently has sufficient material been available for widespread testing.

Paclitaxel functions unlike any known agent. It binds to the material that makes up the spindle during M phase of the cell cycle. The spindle is the apparatus that aligns and draws the chromosomes into the two daughter cells. Paclitaxel binds to the spindle, freezing it, and thereby blocking the cell from dividing.

Paclitaxel was approved by the FDA only recently, so the full scope of the tumors against which it is active is not known. However, it has shown activity in a number of solid tumors, and is used in combination with other agents to treat ovarian cancer, lung cancer, cancer of the stomach, leukemia, breast cancer. The FDA expedited approval of Paclitaxel because of the surprising high response rate in patients with ovarian cancer who had become resistant to the standard drugs.

Paclitaxel is given intravenously by a slow infusion over 24 hours.

SIDE EFFECTS

- Many patients have an immediate allergic reaction to Paclitaxel. This reaction can range from swelling, especially around the throat, to flushed skin which may develop into a rash. These effects can be reduced by giving the drug over a long infusion and treatment with corticosteroids.
- Bone marrow toxicity (myelosuppression) is the most common side effect of Paclitaxel. This is a side effect of killing the stem cells in your bone marrow that produce new blood cells. It is detected when the cells in your blood are counted. The laboratory typically finds a reduction in white cells (neutropenia). The lowest counts are usually seen about 10 days after the drug was given. Your white cell counts will return to normal about 5 days after this.
- Hair loss is a frequent side effect, but usually reverses. Hair loss (called alopecia) does not threaten your health, but it can have a profound affect on how you feel about yourself. Many patients find the changes to their appearance, such as alopecia or changes in their fingernails, more devastating than the events that are more significant from a medical point of view.
- Nausea and vomiting (emesis) are common side effects of Paclitaxel. Even with combinations of corticosteroids and the new anti-emetic drugs, many patients still have terrible nausea.
- Other effects on the digestive system include diarrhea and intestinal bleeding.
- Mouth sores (stomatitis) are common and very unpleasant side effects. They are extremely painful, and affect your ability to swallow. It is important to keep your mouth clean and moist until this condition goes away.
- Flushing of the skin, and sometimes rashes on the palms, soles of the feet, chest and neck are reported.
- Flu-like symptoms are often reported, including fever, pain in your muscles and bone, and just feeling very sick (malaise).

- Nerve damage, which usually (but doesn't always) go away after a few months, is known to happen, especially with large doses. This is detected as numbness or tingling, pain (especially in the feet), loss of coordination that may make walking more difficult than normal.

Pentostatin

Pentostatin is an antibiotic originally discovered from soil samples. Bacteria living in soil have evolved ways to produce many noxious compounds to help them compete with other bacteria that share their habitat. Pharmaceutical companies have been systematically collecting soil samples from around the world for years, and many of our most important antibiotics have come from different members of this bacterial family called Streptomyces. Pentostatin is also known as 2-Deoxycoformycin, dCF or by its brand name Nipent® (Parke Davis).

Pentostatin is similar in structure to the natural cell component, adenosine, and works by "tricking" cell enzymes that operate on adenosine to block cell growth. The particular enzyme that is most susceptible is called "adenosine deaminase" or ADA, although other enzymes are fooled as well. By blocking these enzymes, Pentostatin prevents cells from growing normally.

Cells rich in ADA are selective targets of Pentostatin. These include lymphocytes and malignancies of lymphocytes, including hairy cell leukemia, T-cell leukemia, and lymphoblastic leukemia.

Pentostatin is given into the vein slowly, over 30 minutes.

SIDE EFFECTS

- Kidney damage (nephrotoxicity) can be life threatening, and is the most common reason for limiting or stopping the dose of Pentostatin. Doctors have learned that giving fluids to increase flow through the kidneys before dosing helps protect them, so it has become routine practice.
- Bone marrow toxicity (myelosuppression) can be so severe in some patients it limits the amount of Pentostatin they can tolerate. Usually these are patients whose marrow has been depleted by prior treatment. This is a side effect of killing the stem cells in your bone marrow that produce new blood cells. It is detected when the cells in your blood are counted. The laboratory typically finds a reduction in white cells (neutropenia). The lowest counts are usually seen around day 15 after the drug was given. Your white cell counts will return to normal 10 days after this. Platelet reduction (thrombocytopenia) is seen, too.
- Depletion of lymphocytes is expected, and the lack of lymphocytes makes patients especially sensitive to fever and infections with pneumonia, fungi or viruses are common.
- Neurologic toxicity is detected as fatigue and lethargy. Occasionally seizures occur at high doses.
- Nausea and vomiting (emesis) are usually mild and not a major concern.
- Other effects on the digestive system include diarrhea and intestinal bleeding.
- Dry skin is frequently reported, which occasionally is accompanied with a rash. Also, patients may be susceptible to viral infections such as Herpes.

- Eye irritation (conjunctivitis) can be a problem for some patients. Eyedrops containing a drug like dexamethasone help control this. This condition will go away in time.

Pentoxifylline

Pentoxyfylline, or Trental® (Hoechst Marion Roussel), is not an anti-cancer drug, but a drug used to control some of the side effects of treatment. It is approved for facilitating blood flow in patients with diseases that affect the peripheral vasculature.

Pentoxifilline is believed to reduce the production of an important signal molecule secreted by macrophages, TNF-α. This signal molecule is produced in reaction to certain stressful situations as your body mounts its defense. It is known to cause some of the side effects in cancer and its treatment, such as weight loss. It is being tested in experimental trials in cancer patients, to help lower the severity of mucositis, weight loss and reduce the hospital stay. It is not certain yet whether it is effective.

SIDE EFFECTS

- Pentoxyfylline is generally well tolerated, and has been used in Europe since 1972. However, some side effects have been noted as follows:
- Affects on the nervous system include dizziness, headache and insomnia.
- Some patients experience mild stomach upset, indigestion, flatulence or nausea.
- Affects on the cardiovascular system can include chest pains, swelling (edema) and lowered blood pressure.

PIXY-321

PIXY-321 is prepared by chemical joining of two biological proteins, Interleukin-3 and the Growth Control Signal that regulates the rate of production of granulocytes and macrophages (GM-CSF).

PIXY-321 is not an anti-cancer agent, but is designed to stimulate the repopulation of the bone marrow to control myelosuppression, similar to GM-CSF and G-CSF. The rationale for splicing the two together came from observations that, used separately, IL-3 and GM-CSF seemed to make each other more powerful in replenishing stem cells in the marrow.

PIXY-321 is an experimental agent presently under evaluation in clinical trials. Data from these trials suggest that perhaps PIXY-321 helps replenish platelets as well as neutrophils, although this has not been proven as yet.

PIXY-321 is given by injection just beneath the skin.

SIDE EFFECTS

- To date the major side effect is a reddening of the skin at the site of injection. More information about side effects will come out as the trials progress.

Prednisone

Prednisone, also known as Dehydrocortisone, (Pharmacia and Upjohn's brand-name is Deltasone®, and there are many others) is a synthetic imitation of the natural hormones Cortisone and Hydroxycortisone. It is not an anti-cancer drug, but helps overcome some of the side effects of cancer and cancer treatments. It is frequently given after Cisplatin chemotherapy to help manage the debilitating effects of platinum compounds on fatigue and the patients' sense of well being.

Cortisone, Hydrocortisone and Prednisone are members of a family of very active biological molecules called glucocorticoids. The former two are signal molecules that regulate a number of different biological functions. Prednisone was designed to duplicate the anti-inflammatory activity, but have less affect on other functions. In particular, use of cortisone stimulates the adrenals to alter the water-retention balance. Prednisone doesn't stimulate this action as much, so has less of these side effects.

Patients on Prednisone should avoid stressful situations as much as possible, since some of the physiological responses to stress are regulated by the adrenal cortex, and will not function as effectively. Also, there is an increased risk of developing yeast infections for patients on Prednisone.

SIDE EFFECTS

- Fluid retention. While this side effect is less noticeable than cortisone, it is not eliminated completely.
- Increased blood pressure (hypertension) can result from prednisone use, and congestive heart failure is a risk in susceptible patients.
- Muscle effects, including weakness, wasting away of muscle is known to occur in some patients.
- Loss of bone (osteoporosis) can result from Prednisone use, which increases your susceptibility to bone fractures.
- Effects on the stomach and gastrointestinal system can include developing ulcers, and/or inflammation of the esophagus.
- The central nervous system can be affected, causing dizziness, headaches, and sometimes convulsions.
- The menstrual cycle may be affected, causing irregularities, since glucocorticoids are similar to estrogen.

Procarbazine

Procarbazine, or Matulane® (Roche) is a small synthetic compound that has been available for many years.

Procarbazine is activated inside cells to form several different alkylating agents that bind to DNA and prevent cell growth. The exact mechanism of how this works is not understood, because of the number and complexity of the reactions. We do know that the result is to break chromosomes and block production of new DNA.

Procarbazine is used primarily to treat Hodgkin's Disease, a form of lymphoma, in a combination with other anti-cancer drugs. The demonstration that a combination of agents known as MOPP in 1970 completely led to a high cure rate for this disease was a watershed in treatment of cancer with chemical therapies. Procarbazine is one of the two "Ps" in MOPP, with Prednisone. It is sometimes used to treat cancer of the brain and small cell lung cancer.

Procarbazine is usually given orally, as a capsule.

SIDE EFFECTS

- Bone marrow toxicity (myelosuppression) is the most common side effect of Procarbazine. This is a side effect of killing the stem cells in your bone marrow that produce new blood cells. It is detected when the cells in your blood are counted. The laboratory typically finds a reduction in platelets (thrombocytopenia). The lowest counts are usually seen about 4 weeks after the drug was given.
- At higher doses, the myelosuppressive effects extend to other blood cells, and limit the amount of drug you can tolerate.
- Nausea and vomiting (emesis) are common side effects of Procarbazine, but are not usually severe..
- Other effects on the digestive system include diarrhea and intestinal bleeding.
- Flu-like symptoms are often reported, including fever, chills, pain in your muscles and bone, and just feeling very sick (malaise). These usually are limited to the first dose.
- Effects on the central nervous system happen to about one in three patients, and can be disturbing. These effects may include nightmares, depression and insomnia or even hallucinations. Other symptoms are lack of coordination, dizziness or headaches.

Sargramostim (GM-CSF)

Sargramostim is a genetic engineering product that is designed to mimic the natural growth control signal that triggers production of the stem cells that produce granulocytes and monocytes. It also is known as Granulocyte Macrophage - Colony Stimulating Factor (GM-CSF), and is available in from two sources: Leukine® (Immunex) and Prokine® (Hoechst Marion Roussel) is produced from yeast cells, while Leukomax® (Schering) is produced from bacteria. Another version, produced in cultured hamster cells, was never marketed.

GM-CSF is not an anti-cancer drug, but helps manage the recovery of bone marrow after chemotherapy or radiation. Within the marrow, a series of partially differentiated stem cells are poised to replace your body's white cells depending on the needs. One stem cell that is intermediate in the maturation pathway is designed to respond to a growth control signal, Sargramostim. When triggered, that cell begins to multiply and the daughters mature further, the net effect of which is to increase the number of monocytes and granulocytes in the blood.

GM-CSF, like PIXY-321 and G-CSF, is used to hasten the recovery of your white blood cells. The range of procedures are explained further in the section on Stem Cell Support.

Sargramostim is given by injection, either just under the skin, or into a vein in an infusion.

SIDE EFFECTS

- At low doses, the most frequent side effect is a flu-like syndrome, sometimes accompanied by headaches. You might feel lethargic, or just plain miserable (malaise). These symptoms usually go away in a few hours.
- Sometimes the first dose causes an effect on the cardiovascular system, such as lowered blood pressure, and shortness of breath.
- Pain in your bones is often reported. It feels like a dull ache, especially in your long bones.
- A local irritation at the site of injection may develop.
- At high doses the side effects may be severe. The walls of your capillaries may loosen, allowing fluid to leak out and dropping your blood pressure. Your lungs may start to fill with fluid and the lining of the chest cavity may become inflamed.

Tamoxifen

The brand name of Tamoxifen is Nolvadex® (Zeneca). It is a synthetic compound designed to mimic the signal hormone estrogen.

Estrogen, like many signal hormones, is produced at one site (the ovaries) whence it circulates to the organs that need to respond to the signal. Among the many estrogen responsive cells are those in the breasts, which prepare for the potential pregnancy during the menstrual cycle. This response by the cells occurs because there is an estrogen receptor on them, to which the estrogen binds, which event then triggers a series of changes in cell activity.

The daughters of the cell that initiated the tumor in breast cancer will have estrogen receptors in about two thirds of patients. Years ago it was common to remove the ovaries from women with breast cancer, because the cancer cells stopped growing when the estrogen was removed. Now we duplicate this effect by treating with Tamoxifen, which ties up the estrogen receptors so they can't respond to estrogen.

Tamoxifen is given orally as a tablet.

SIDE EFFECTS

- Tamoxifen is relatively non-toxic, especially in women who have undergone menopause.
- However, it does neutralize many estrogen activities. It can induce menopause symptoms in premenopausal patients. It may affect the menstrual cycle, such as increased bleeding. It can cause skin rashes, depression or headaches. It may also increase water retention, and affect your taste for food.

Taxotere

Taxotere, or dexetaxel, is a compound of the Taxane family recently approved by the FDA. It is a partially synthetic molecule designed to mimic Paclitaxel.

Like Paclitaxel it binds to the material that makes up the spindle during M phase of the cell cycle. The spindle is the apparatus that aligns and draws the chromosomes into the two daughter cells in the M phase of the Cell Cycle. Taxotere binds to the spindle, freezing it, and thereby blocks the cell from dividing.

The range of tumors against which it is active are only now being reported.

Taxotere is given by injection into the vein over about an hour infusion.

SIDE EFFECTS

- Many patients have an immediate allergic reaction to Taxotere. This reaction can range from swelling, especially around the throat, to flushed skin which may develop into a rash. These effects can be reduced by giving the drug over a long infusion and treatment with corticosteroids.
- Bone marrow toxicity (myelosuppression) is the most common side effect of Taxotere. This is a side effect of killing the stem cells in your bone marrow that produce new blood cells. It is detected when the cells in your blood are counted. The laboratory typically finds a reduction in white cells (neutropenia).
- Hair loss is a frequent side effect, but usually reverses. Hair loss (called alopecia) does not threaten your health, but it can have a profound affect on how you feel about yourself. Many patients find the changes to their appearance, such as alopecia or changes in their fingernails, more devastating than the events that are more significant from a medical point of view.
- Flushing of the skin, and sometimes rashes on the palms, soles of the feet, chest and neck are reported.
- Swelling of the limbs which may cause your lungs to fill with fluid are another form of toxicity seen with Taxotere (edema).

Teniposide

Teniposide is also known by the brand name Vumon® (Bristol-Myers Oncology). Like etoposide, it is a chemically modified version of a compound isolated from the mandrake root (also known as the May apple).

Teniposide is an experimental drug not yet approved. Like its well known cousin, it derives from folk medicine, as pharmaceutical companies isolate and study the compounds present in the plants used in old recipes. The medicinal properties of the European mandrake root is mentioned in the Bible, and is referred to in formularies throughout European history.

We believe the compound works through blocking the action of the topoisomerase enzymes. These enzymes are necessary for managing the twisting and coiling of the DNA that takes place when the cell is getting ready to reproduce. When Teniposide is used on cells in the laboratory, they cannot divide and the DNA is found fragmented in pieces bound with to proteins.

Teniposide is administered intravenously.

SIDE EFFECTS

- Bone marrow. The primary toxicity of Teniposide is that it kills the stem cells in your bone marrow that produce new blood cells. This toxicity is detected when the cells in your blood are counted. The laboratory typically finds a reduction in white cells (neutropenia) and platelets (thrombocyto-penia). The lowest counts happen about 7 days after the drug was given. Bone marrow toxicity is temporary, since not all the stem cells are killed, and your white cell counts will return to normal 22 days after the drug is given.
- Nausea and vomiting (emesis) are also reported occasionally.
- Kidney or liver function is not usually a problem except in patients whose organs are impaired. These are likely to have that condition worsened by Teniposide.
- Headaches and fever are common.
- Toxic effects that happen in a small proportion of patients receiving tenoposide include mouth sores (mucositis), allergic reactions, wheezing, and skin lesions. Less than 3% of patients become terribly tired and sleepy as a result of the drug's effect on the nervous system.
- Leukemia. As with many anti-cancer drugs, there is concern that the drugs used to treat cancer can cause a second type of cancer, like leukemia, to develop.

Thioguanine

Thioguanine, 6-TG of Tabloid® (Glaxo-Wellcome) is a small synthetic molecule designed to imitate the natural product, hypoxanthine, which is used to make some components of DNA.

It is classified as an antimetabolite, similar to 6-Mercaptopurine, or Pentostatin. It must be activated inside the cell by fooling some of the enzymes used to produce DNA.

It interferes with several biochemical pathways to kill the cell, including DNA and RNA synthesis.

It is active against several forms of leukemia. One important difference between it and 6-Mercaptopurine is that Thioguanine may be given together with Allupurinol.

Thioguanine is given orally as a tablet.

SIDE EFFECTS

- Bone marrow toxicity (myelosuppression) is the most common side effect of 6-Mercaptopurine, but is not severe at the normal doses. This is a side effect of killing the stem cells in your bone marrow that produce new blood cells. It is detected when the cells in your blood are counted. The laboratory typically finds a reduction in white cells (neutropenia) and platelets (thrombocytopenia). The lowest counts are usually seen between day 11 and 23 after the drug was given. Your white cell counts will return to normal 10 days after this.
- Nausea and vomiting (emesis) are uncommon side effects of Thioguanine.
- Other rare effects on the digestive system include severe diarrhea and intestinal bleeding.
- Mouth sores (stomatitis) are common and very unpleasant side effects. They are extremely painful, and affect your ability to swallow. It is important to keep your mouth clean and moist until this condition goes away.
- Liver damage has been observed in a few patients, so is considered possible. It can be severe in a few instances.
- Blood in the urine is sometimes seen with high doses. Other effects on the kidney may be related to the presence of crystals of Thioguanine, which can interrupt flow and cause serious nephrotoxicity.

Thiotepa

Thiotepa is a small synthetic compound that binds to DNA and proteins to block cell replication.

It is not used as frequently as other alkylating agents except in topical uses, such as papillary tumors of the bladder. In combination with other drugs it is used to treat cancers of the breast, bladder and ovaries, Hodgkin's disease and it is used to stimulate the marrow in bone marrow transplantation.

Thiotepa is given by injection, either into a vein or into a cavity such as the bladder, heart or lung cavity.

SIDE EFFECTS

- Bone marrow toxicity (myelosuppression) is the most common side effect of Thiotepa. This is a side effect of killing the stem cells in your bone marrow that produce new blood cells. It is detected when the cells in your blood are counted. The laboratory typically finds a reduction in white cells (neutropenia). The lowest counts are usually seen between day 7 and 10 after the drug was given. Platelet counts will go down (thrombocytopenia), if at all, after this.

- Nausea and vomiting (emesis) are common side effects of Thiotepa.

Topotecan

Topotecan, or Hycamtin® (SmithKline Beecham) was recently approved by the FDA. It is produced by modifying a compound that is extracted from a tree found in China. The natural product, camptothecin, is another in the long list of folk medicines which contain an active compound when analyzed by scientists. Camptothecin proved too toxic when tested in clinical trials, so modifications have been made. Topotecan and CPT-11 are both derived from this compound.

All three compounds work by blocking the topoisomerase enzymes, which prevents the cell from duplicating its DNA. These enzymes, described in the section on Chromosomes, help manage the supercoiled DNA during replication. Once bound, Topotecan prevents cells from copying the DNA.

Toptecan is actvie against several types of cancer, including lung and ovarian cancer. It is administered by intravenous infusion.

SIDE EFFECTS

- Toxicity to the Bone marrow (myelosuppression) is the most severe side effect with Topotecan.
- Nausea and vomiting (emesis).
- Hair loss is a frequent side effect, but usually reverses. Hair loss (called alopecia) does not threaten your health, but it can have a profound affect on how you feel about yourself.
- Many patients find the changes to their appearance, such as alopecia or changes in their fingernails, more devastating than the events that are more significant from a medical point of view.

Tretinoin

Tretinoin is also known as ATRA, or All *trans* Retinoic Acid. Normally, Vitamin A (Retinol) is made by the liver out of ß-carotene in your diet. Retinol is present in the blood, but is changed into retinoic acid once it gets inside cells. Providing Tretinoin as a drug directly bypasses the natural pathway described above.

Tretinoin is a genetic signal molecule. That is, it interacts directly with DNA to turn on a series of genes that affect the cell's behavior. We don't fully understand the purpose of all of these genes, but we do know that Tretinoin stops cells from dividing and causes them to mature. For some cancers, this pushes them out of the cell cycle and forces them further down the maturation pathway they began before they lost control.

Tretinoin approved by the FDA. It has proven to be active in one form of leukemia, but it is not certain whether it will have broader use. Because it works differently than most anti-cancer drugs its progress is being watched carefully.

Tretinoin is usually administered orally, as a capsule. An injectable form in liposomes is also being studied.

SIDE EFFECTS

- The most common side effect is headaches, which are usually manageable. Severe headaches may be due to high pressure on the brain, and require lumbar puncture and corticosteroid treatment.
- Tretinoin produces dry skin and mucous membranes, which may turn red, slough off and develop into sores, especially on the lips.
- Bone pain can be intense but is controlled with analgesics.
- Lung toxicity, including fluid in the lungs, high fever and infiltration of fluid into the heart cavity are called the "Retinoic Acid Syndrome." It may require use of a ventilator, even inserting tubes into the trachea to maintain oxygen flow. Corticosteroids appear to prevent this condition.
- Tretinoin causes birth defects, and must not be given to pregnant women.

Vinblastine

Vinblastine is also known as VLB or by its brand name of Velban® (Lilly). It is produced by the ornamental flowering vine, periwinkle (*Vinca rosa*). Vinblastine and its cousin Vincristine are more examples of an effective medicine that was produced by examining the ingredients in folk medicine. Another name for periwinkle is dog bane, which has been used in many herbal potions for centuries.

The Vinca alkaloids Vinblastine and Vincristine work by preventing the spindle from forming, which blocks the cells' ability to divide. The spindle is the apparatus that aligns and draws the chromosomes into the two daughter cells during the M phase of the Cell Cycle.

Vinblastine is effective alone, but is most often used as part of a combination therapy with other anti-cancer drugs. It is used against lymphomas, testicular, lung and breast cancer as well as others.

Vinblastine is given by injection into the vein.

SIDE EFFECTS

- Vinblastine causes a severe reaction to tissues it comes in contact with. Great care should be taken to make sure it all goes into the vein at the site of injection.
- Bone marrow toxicity (myelosuppression) is the most common side effect of Vinblastine. This is a side effect of killing the stem cells in your bone marrow that produce new blood cells. It is detected when the cells in your blood are counted. The laboratory typically finds a reduction in white cells (neutropenia). The lowest counts are usually seen between day 4 and 10 after the drug was given. Your white cell counts will return to normal 2 weeks after this. Platelet reduction (thrombocytopenia) is not as common and is not severe.

- Hair loss is a frequent side effect, but usually reverses. Hair loss (called alopecia) does not threaten your health, but it can have a profound affect on how you feel about yourself. Many patients find the changes to their appearance, such as alopecia or changes in their fingernails, more devastating than the events that are more significant from a medical point of view.
- Nausea and vomiting (emesis) are not as serious as with other anti-cancer drugs
- Other effects on the digestive system include constipation and stomach cramps.
- Mouth sores (stomatitis) are very unpleasant side effects. They are extremely painful, and affect your ability to swallow. It is important to keep your mouth clean and moist until this condition goes away.
- Liver damage is a potential side effect, although not common. This would show up in laboratory tests of your blood, and will go away spontaneously.
- Flushing of the skin, and sometimes rashes are reported.
- Nerve damage, which usually (but doesn't always) go away, is known to happen, especially with large doses. This could show up as numbness, depression, or headaches.

Vincristine (Oncovin)

Vincristine is also known as VCR or by its brand name of Oncovin® (Lilly). It is produced by the ornamental flowering vine, periwinkle (*Vinca rosa*). Vincristine and its cousins Vinblastine and Vindesine are more examples of an effective medicine that was produced by examining the ingredients in folk medicine. Another name for periwinkle is dog bane, which has been used in many herbal potions for centuries.

The Vinca alkaloids Vincristine and Vinblastine work by preventing the spindle from forming, which blocks the cells' ability to divide. The spindle is the apparatus that aligns and draws the chromosomes into the two daughter cells during the M phase of the Cell Cycle. Although produced by the same plant, the two behave differently and are used in different settings.

Vincristine is effective alone, but is most often used as part of a combination therapy with other anti-cancer drugs. It is used against leukemia, lymphoma and breast cancer as well as others.

Vincristine is given by injection into the vein. This can be rapid, or by a slow infusion over several days.

SIDE EFFECTS

- Vincristine causes a severe reaction to tissues it comes in contact with. Great care should be taken to make sure it all goes into the vein at the site of injection.
- Nerve damage, in the form of jaw pain, numbness in the extremities and muscle weakness is the most common side effect with Vincristine. Fever, fatigue and anorexia may evolve a day or so after dosing.
- Bone marrow toxicity (myelosuppression) is less severe than with Vinblastine, and as a result is used more often in combinations with other drugs that are toxic to the bone marrow.

- Nausea and vomiting (emesis) are not as serious as with other anti-cancer drugs, but constipation and stomach pain can be very uncomfortable.
- Mouth sores (stomatitis) are very unpleasant side effects. They are extremely painful, and affect your ability to swallow. It is important to keep your mouth clean and moist until this condition goes away.
- Liver damage is a potential side effect, although not common. This would show up in laboratory tests of your blood, and will go away spontaneously.
- Flushing of the skin, and sometimes rashes are reported.

Vindesine

Vindesine is also known as Eldisine or DVA. It is a chemically modified version of Vinblastine, which is produced by the ornamental flowering vine, periwinkle (*Vinca rosa*). Vinblastine and its cousin Vincristine are more examples of an effective medicine that was produced by examining the ingredients in folk medicine. Another name for periwinkle is dog bane, which has been used in many herbal potions for centuries.

The Vinca alkaloids Vinblastine and Vincristine work by preventing the spindle from forming, which blocks the cells' ability to divide. The spindle is the apparatus that aligns and draws the chromosomes into the two daughter cells during the M phase of the Cell Cycle. Vindesine was produced to overcome some of the known problems with Vinblastine.

Vindesine is an experimental drug not yet approved by the FDA. It is effective alone, but is most often studied as part of a combination therapy with other anti-cancer drugs. It is being studied most often against lung cancer, where it has shown some success, but is also being studied against other types of cancer.

Vindesine is given by injection into the vein.

SIDE EFFECTS

- Bone marrow toxicity (myelosuppression) is the most common side effect of Vindesine. This is a side effect of killing the stem cells in your bone marrow that produce new blood cells. It is detected when the cells in your blood are counted. The laboratory typically finds a reduction in white cells (neutropenia). The lowest counts are usually seen between day 4 and 10 after the drug was given. Your white cell counts will return to normal 2 weeks after this. Platelet reduction (thrombocytopenia) is not as common and is not severe.
- Nerve damage, in the form of jaw pain, numbness in the extremities and muscle weakness is common with Vindesine. Fever, fatigue and anorexia may evolve a day or so after dosing.
- Hair loss is a frequent side effect, but usually reverses. Hair loss (called alopecia) does not threaten your health, but it can have a profound affect on how you feel about yourself.
- Many patients find the changes to their appearance, such as alopecia or changes in their fingernails, more devastating than the events that are more significant from a medical point of view.
- Nausea and vomiting (emesis) are not as serious as with other anti-cancer drugs

- Other effects on the digestive system include constipation and stomach cramps.
- Mouth sores (stomatitis) are very unpleasant side effects. They are extremely painful, and affect your ability to swallow. It is important to keep your mouth clean and moist until this condition goes away.

Vinorelbine (Navelbine)

Vinorelbine is also known as Navelbine® (Glaxo Wellcome). It is a chemically modified version of Vinblastine, which is produced by the ornamental flowering vine, periwinkle (*Vinca rosa*). Vinblastine and its cousin Vincristine are examples of an effective medicine that was produced by examining the ingredients in folk medicine. Another name for periwinkle is dog bane, which has been used in many herbal potions for centuries.

The Vinca alkaloids Vinblastine and Vincristine work by preventing the spindle from forming, which blocks the cells' ability to divide. The spindle is the apparatus that aligns and draws the chromosomes into the two daughter cells during the M phase of the Cell Cycle. Vinorelbine was produced to overcome some of the known problems with Vinblastine.

Vinorelbine was just approved by the FDA. It is effective alone, but is most often studied as part of a combination therapy with other anti-cancer drugs. It is being studied most often against breast and lung cancer, where it has shown some success, but is also being studied against other types of cancer.

Vinorelbine is given by injection into the vein or as a capsule.

SIDE EFFECTS

- Bone marrow toxicity (myelosuppression) is the most common side effect of Vindesine. This is a side effect of killing the stem cells in your bone marrow that produce new blood cells. It is detected when the cells in your blood are counted. The laboratory typically finds a reduction in white cells (neutropenia). The lowest counts are usually seen between day 4 and 10 after the drug was given. Your white cell counts will return to normal a week after this. Anemia is also reported.
- Nerve damage, in the form of numbness in the extremities and muscle weakness is common with Vinorelbine.
- Hair loss (alopecia) is not common in patients who take Vinorelbine. Your hair will grow back, but it is disturbing to some.
- Nausea and vomiting (emesis) are not as serious as with other anti-cancer drugs

CLINICAL ASSESSMENTS OF TOXICITY

Evaluating Patients' Overall health.

One of the pioneers in developing chemotherapy as a means of treating cancer in the 1940s was Dr. David Karnofsky. Among his many contributions, he developed the following scale for classifying the health status of patients. It is used in many clinical trials, and is provided for you if you are reading about them. As you see, it classifies patients' overall health into ten categories as follows:

Karnofsky Performance Scale

Score	Description	Score	Description
100	Normal; no complaints; no evidence of disease	40	Disabled; requires special care and assistance
90	Able to carry on normal activity; minor signs or symptoms of disease	30	Severely disabled; hospitalization indicated. Death not imminent
80	Normal activity with effort; some signs or symptoms of disease	20	Very sick; hospitalization necessary; active support treatment necessary
70	Cares for self; unable to carry on normal activity or to do active work	10	Moribund; fatal process; progressing rapidly
60	Requires occasional assistance, but is able to care for most of his/her needs	0	Dead
50	Requires considerable assistance and frequent medical care		

EVALUATING THE SEVERITY OF TOXICITY

There are many tests available to help assess your health. Some are done by drawing blood, or urine and checking to see whether the amount of different markers are within normal range. Abnormal values may be very significant to your health, or they may be expected for your condition. Your physician is in the best position to interpret the test results.

The National Cancer Institute developed a systematic method for grading the severity of toxicity for most organ functions. It is called the NCI Common Toxicity scale, and is presented in the next few pages. Using this scale, the results from different hospitals across the country can be compared.

This information is provided to help you put into perspective some of the results from your laboratory tests. You should understand that the people who are in the best position to evaluate the significance of these tests is your team of care givers, and be sure to consult with them about any concerns you may have before making judgments about your condition. It is very easy to jump to the wrong conclusion in reading test results.

Grade 1 Toxicity is sometimes called Mild Toxicity, Grade 2 Moderate, Grade 3 Moderately Severe, and Grade 4 Severe.

Different hospital laboratories vary a little in the range of results they get for some tests. To account for this, you will see values in these tables expressed as "1.5 times the upper normal." This means the test result is 50% higher than the highest result that is considered normal for that particular test in that laboratory. For example, let's say your hospital normally finds bilirubin values between 0.2 and 1.5 mg/dL in healthy individuals. The upper normal is 1.5, so a value of 2.25 mg/dL would be 1.5 times the upper normal. Anything above that would be considered Grade 2 toxicity.

GRADING SEVERE AND MODERATE TOXIC EFFECTS

ITEM	GRADE 1 TOXICITY	GRADE 2 TOXICITY	GRADE 3 TOXICITY	GRADE 4 TOXICITY
HEMATOLOGY				
Hemoglobin	9.5-10.5 g/dl	8.0-9.4 g/dl	6.5-7.9 g/dl	<6.5 g/dl
Absolute Neutrophil Count	$1000\text{-}1500/mm^3$	$750\text{-}999/mm^3$	$500\text{-}749 \ mm^3$	$<500/mm^3$
Platelets	$75\text{ -}99,000/mm^3$	$50\text{ -}74,999/mm^3$	$20\text{ -}49,999/mm^3$	$<20,000/mm^3$ or diffuse petechiae
PT	1.01-1.25 X upper normal 1.01-1.66 X upper normal	1.26-1.5 X upper normal 1.67-2.33 X upper normal	1.51-3.0 X upper normal 2.34-3 X upper normal	>3 X upper normal >3 X upper normal
PTT	0.74-0.50 X lower normal	0.74-0.50 X lower normal	0.49-0.25 X lower normal	<0.24 X lower normal
Fibrinogen	20-40 µg/ml	41-50 µg/ml	51-60 µg/ml	>60 µg/ml
Fibrin Split Product	5-9.9%	10.0-14.9%	15.0-19.9%	>20%
Met-hemoglobin	None	None	None	None
SERUM CHEMISTRY				
Hyponatremia	130-135 meq/L	123-129 meq/L	116-122 meq/L	115 meq/L and less *or* mental status changes or seizures
Hypernatremia	146-150 meq/L	151-157 meq/L	158-165 meq/L	>165 meq/L or mental status changes or seizures
Hypokalemia	3.0-3.4 meq/L	2.5-2.9 meq/L or replacement Rx req.	2.0-2.4 meq/L or intensive replacement Rx Reg. or Hosp.	< 2. meq/L or paresis or ileus or life-threatening arrhythmia
Hyperkalemia	5.6-6.0 meq/L	6.1-6.5 meq/L	6.6-7.0 meq/L	>7.0 or paresis or ileus or life-threatening arrhythmia

ITEM	GRADE 1 TOXICITY	GRADE 2 TOXICITY	GRADE 3 TOXICITY	GRADE 4 TOXICITY
CHEMISTRIES				
Hypoglycemia	55-64 mg/dl	40-54 mg/dl	30-39 mg/dl	<30 mg/dl or mental status changes or coma
Hyperglycemia	116-160 mg/dl	161-250 mg/dl	251-500 mg/dl	>500 mg/dl or ketoacidosis or seizures
Hypertriglyceridemia	< 399 mg/dl	400-999 mg/dl	>1,000 mg/dl	
Hyperuricemia	7.5-9.9 mg/dl	10.0-12.0 mg/dl	12.1-15.0 mg/dl	>15.0 mg/dl
Hypocalcemia correct for albumin	8.4-7.8 mg/dl	7.7-7.0 mg/dl	6.9-6.1 mg/dl	<6.1 mg/dl or life threatening arrhythmia or tetanus
Hypercalcemia correct for albumin	10.6-11.5 mg/dl	11.6 - 12.5 mg/dl	12.6 - 13.5 mg/dl	>13.5 mg/dl or tetany or life-threatening arrhythmia
Hypomagnesia	1.4-1.2 meq/L	1.1-0.9 meq/L or replacement Rx req.	0.8-0.6 meq/L or intensive Rx req. hospitalization	<0.6 meq/L or life threatening arrhythmia's
Phosphate	2.0-2.4	1.5-1.9 or replacement Rx req.	1.0-1.4 meq/L intensive Rx req. hospitalization	<1.0 life-threatening arrhythmia's or
Bilirubin (Liver)	1-1.5 x upper normal	1.6-2.5 x upper normal	2.6-5 x upper normal	>5 x upper normal
Blood Urea Nitrogen (Kidney)	1.26-2.5 x upper normal	2.6-5 X upper normal	5.1-10 x upper normal	>10 x upper normal
Creatinine (Kidney)	0.5-1.5 x upper normal	1.6-3 x upper normal	3.1-6 x upper normal	>6 x upper normal or requires dialysis
SERUM ENZYMES				
AST (SGOT) (Liver)	1.26-2.5 x upper normal	2.6-5 x upper normal	5.1-10 x upper normal	>10 x upper normal
ALT (SGPT) (Liver)	1.25-2.5 x upper normal	2.6-5 x upper normal	5.1-10 x upper normal	>10 x upper normal
GGT (Liver)	1.25-2.5 x upper normal	2.6-5 x upper normal	5.1-10 x upper normal	>10 x upper normal
ALKALINE PHOSPHATASE (Liver)	1.25-2.5 x upper normal	2.6-5 x upper normal	5.1-10 x upper normal	>10 x upper normal
AMYLASE (Pancreas)	1.1-1.5 x upper normal	1.6--2.0 x upper normal	2,1-5.0 x upper normal, mild clinical pancreatitis	5.1 x normal or severe clinical pancreatitis

ITEM	GRADE 1 TOXICITY	GRADE 2 TOXICITY	GRADE 3 TOXICITY	GRADE 4 TOXICITY
URINALYSIS				
Proteinuria	1+ or <0.03% or g/L or 200 mg/lg loss/day	2-3+ or 0..3-1.0% or 3-10 g/L 1-2 g loss/day	4+ or >1.0% or >10 g/L 2-3.5 g loss/day	nephrotic syndrome or >3.5 g loss/day
Hematuria	microscopic only <10	gross, no clots, 11-100	gross + clots,>101	obstructive or req.
CARDIAC				
Cardiac Rhythm	asymptomatic, transient signs, no Rx required	recurrent/ persistent no Rx required	requires treatment	requires monitoring or hypotension or ventricular tachycardia or fibrillation hospitalization
Hypertension	transient > 20 mm no Rx	recurrent, chronic >20 mm, Rx req.	requires outpt. acute Rx	
Hypotension	transient orthostatic hypotension, No Rx	symptoms correctable with oral fluid Rx	requires IV fluids no hosp. required	requires hospitalization
Pericarditis	minimal effusion	mild/mod. asymp effusion no Rx	symptomatic effusion, pain EKG changes	tamponade; peri-cardiocentesis or surgery req.
Hemorrhage, Blood Loss	microscopic/ occult	mild, no transfusion	gross blood loss 1-2 units transfused	massive blood loss, >3 units transfused
RESPIRATORY				
COUGH-for aerosol studies	transient-no Rx	treatment assoc. cough, local non-narcotic Rx	treatment assoc. cough, narcotic Rx required	uncontrolled
Shortness of Breath	mild, does not interfere with routine activities	moderate, interferes with routine activities req. intermittent Rx	moderate, debilitating requiring nasal oxygen	severe, requiring ventilator assistance
Bronchospasm Acute	transient, no Rx 70% or peak flow	req. Rx, normalize w/bronchodilator; FEV>50% or peak flow	no normalization w/bronchodilator FEV 25-50% peak flow retraction	cyanosis, FEV <25% or peak flow intubated

ITEM	GRADE 1	GRADE 2	GRADE 3	GRADE 4
DIGESTIVE SYSTEM				
Stomatitis	mild discomfort no limits on activity	some limits on eating/talking	eating/talking very limited	unable to drink fluids; req. IV fluids
Nausea	mild discomfort maintains reasonable intake	mod. discomfort sign dec of intake; some limit of activity	severe discomfort no significant food intake activities limited	hypotensive shock hospitalization IV fluid therapy
Vomiting	transient emesis	occ/moderate vomiting	orthostatic hypotension or IV fluid Rx req.	hypotensive shock hospitalization IV fluid therapy
Constipation	mild	moderate, Rx req.	severe Rx req. vomiting	distention with vomiting
Diarrhea	transient or 3-4 loose stools	5-7 loose stools/day and/ or nocturnal loose stools. Rx req.	orthostatic hypotension of >7 loose stools/day or req. IV fluid Rx	hypotensive shock or hospitalization IV fluid therapy
Abdominal Pain	mild, occasional transient	moderate, transient	severe or req. analgesic	severe with guarding, peritoneal signs
NEURO/NEUROLOGICAL LEVEL OF CONSCIOUSNESS				
Neurocerebellar	slight incoordination Dysdiadokokinesis	intention tremor, dysmetria, slurred speech; nystagmus	locomotor ataxia	incapacitated
Mood	mild anxiety or depression	mod. anxiety or depression and therapy required	severe anxiety or depression or manic; (needs assistance)	acute psychosis; incapacitated req. hospitalization
Neurocontrol	mild anxiety or depression	mod. confusion agitation; some sev. limitation of ADL, min. Rx.	sev. confusion agitation; req. assistance for ADL Rx req.	toxic psychosis; hospitalization
Muscle Strength	subj. weakness; no obj. symptoms/ signs	mild objective no dec. in function	objective weakness function limited	paralysis
Painful Neuropathy	mild discomfort; no therapy req. (any symptom scored 1,2,3 on symptom questionnaire	moderate discomfort persisting for >72 hrs; analgesia req. (any symptom scored 4,5,6 on symptom questionnaire	severe discomfort marked antialgic gait. Narcotic analgesia req. with symptomatic improvement (any symptom scored 7,8,9,10 on symptom questionnaire	incapacitating intolerable discomfort. Not improved unable to walk despite narcotic analges-ics (any symptom scored 7,8,9,10 on symptom questionnaire

ITEM	GRADE 1 TOXICITY	GRADE 2 TOXICITY	GRADE 3 TOXICITY	GRADE 4 TOXICITY
NEUROMUSCULAR				
Myositis	minimal findings	Patients must have some measures of myositis (positive EMG or muscle biopsy) and one of the following	Patients must have some measures of myositis(positive EMG or muscle biopsy) and one of the following:	Patients must have some measures of myositis(positive EMG or muscle biopsy) and one of the following:
		1) mild to moderate myalgias, >4 weeks requiring non-steroidal antiinflammatory agents.	1) moderate/ severe myalgias or muscle tenderness >4 weeks req. non-steroidal anti-inflammatory agents.	1) severe muscle pain (myalgias) not related to exercise, requiring narcotics.
		2) difficulty climbing stairs or rising from a sitting position but able to ambulate without assistance.	2) requires some assistance with ambulation or general activities.	2) muscle weakness resulting in inability to ambulate, req. special care and assistance with mobilization. 3) acute rhabdomyolysis with muscle necrosis and edema, moderate to severe muscle weakness with inability to ambulate or mobilize self without assistance 4) acute rhabdomyolysis associated with electrolyte imbalance or renal failure..

OTHER PARAMETERS				
FEVER oral, W/O infection, >12 hrs	37.7-38.5 °C or 100.0-101.5 °F	38.5-39.5 °C or 101.6-102.8 °F	39.6-40.5 °C or 103-105 °F	>40.5 °C or >105 °F
Headache	mild, no Rx therapy	transient, mod; Rx req.	severe, responds to initial narcotic therapy	intractable, req. repeated narcotic therapy
Fatigue	no dec. in daily activities	normal activity dec. 25-50%	normal activity dec. 50% can't work	unable to care for self
Allergic Reaction	pruritus w/o rash	localized urticaria angioedema	generalized urticaria angioedema	anaphylaxis
Local Reaction	tenderness or erythema	induration <10 cm or phlebitis or inflammation;	induration >10 cm or ulceration	necrosis
Muco-Cutaneous	erythema, pruritus	diffuse, mac. pap rash dry desquamation	vesiculation, moist desquam, ulceration	exfoliative dermatitis, mucous membrane involvement suspected Stevens Johnson or erythema multiform necrosis requiring surgery

SIDE EFFECTS OF SELECTED ANTI-CANCER DRUGS

Key

● Severe, Dose Limiting

◎ Moderate or Occasional

	Heart Damage	Lung Effects	Low White Cells	Low Platelets	Low Red Cells	Nausea	Vomiting	Weight Loss	Mouth Sores	Diarrhea	Constipation	Abdominal Pain	Liver	Kidney	Low Blood Pressure	Nerve Toxicity	Eye Problems	Hypersensitivity	Fever / Flu Symptoms	Hair Loss	Rash	Pigmentation	Nail Malformation	Reproductive Effects	Cancer
Altretamine			◎	◎		◎	●	●		◎		◎	◎	◎		◎				◎	◎				
Bleomycin		●				◎	◎	◎	●				◎	◎				●	◎	◎	●	◎	◎	◎	
Busulfan		●	●	●	●		◎	◎	◎													◎		◎	
Carboplatin			◎	●	◎	◎	◎			◎	◎		◎	◎		◎			◎	◎	◎			◎	◎
Carmustine		◎	●	●		●	◎						◎	◎		◎	◎				◎			◎	◎
Chlorambucil		◎	●	●		◎	◎									◎			◎		◎			◎	◎
Cisplatin	◎		◎	◎	◎	◎	●						◎	●		◎	◎	◎	◎					◎	
Cladribine		●	◎			◎	◎														◎				
CPT-11		●	◎	◎	◎	◎				●										◎	◎				
Cyclophosphamide	◎	◎	●	◎	◎	◎	◎		◎				◎	◎						◎		◎			◎
Cytarabine			◎	●	●	◎	◎	◎	◎	◎	◎		◎			●	◎		◎	◎				◎	
Dacarbazine			◎	◎	◎	●	●						◎		◎					◎	◎				◎
Dactinomycin			●	●	◎	●	◎		●				◎									◎	◎	◎	
Daunorubicin	●		●	◎		◎	◎		◎											◎	◎	◎		◎	
Doxorubicin	●		●	◎	◎	◎	◎		●								◎			◎	◎	◎	◎	◎	◎
Epirubicin	●		●	◎		◎	◎		◎	◎										◎	◎				◎
Etoposide		●	●		◎	◎	◎						◎	◎			◎	◎	◎	◎	◎				◎
Floxuridine		●	◎	◎		◎	◎	●	●		◎	◎		◎						◎	◎	◎	◎		
Fludarabine		◎	●	●	◎	◎	◎			◎		◎	◎			●				◎	◎		◎		
5-Fluorouracil	◎		●	●		◎	◎		●	◎		◎		◎	◎	◎				◎	◎	◎	◎	◎	
Gemcitabine			◎	●	◎	◎	◎												◎		◎				
Idarubicin	●		◎	◎		◎	◎	◎	◎	◎			◎	◎						◎	◎				◎
Ifosfamide		●			◎	◎					◎	●		◎						◎					
Lomustine		◎	●	●	●	◎	◎			◎	◎		◎	◎		◎				◎				◎	◎
Mechlorethamine		●	●	◎	◎	●	●	◎	◎	◎						◎		◎	◎	◎				◎	◎
Melphalan	◎	◎	●	●		◎	◎		◎					◎				◎		◎	◎			◎	◎
6-Mercaptopurine			◎	◎	◎	◎		◎	◎	●			◎	◎					◎		◎				
Methotrexate		◎	●	●	●	◎	◎	◎	●	●			◎	●		◎			◎	◎	◎	◎	◎	◎	
Mitomycin-C		◎	●	●	●	◎	◎		◎	◎			◎	●		◎				◎		◎	◎	◎	
Mitoxantrone	●		●	◎	◎	◎	◎			◎	◎									◎					
Paclitaxel	◎		●	◎	◎	◎	◎		◎	◎		◎		◎	◎	◎		◎	◎	◎	◎				
Pentostatin			●	●		◎	◎			◎			◎	●		●	◎			◎					
Procarbazine		◎	◎	●	●	◎	◎	◎	◎	●					◎	◎	◎	◎	◎	◎	◎			◎	◎
Taxotere		◎	●	◎		◎	◎									◎			◎	◎	◎				
Teniposide			●	●		◎	◎		◎				◎	◎	◎	◎		◎		◎	◎				◎
Thioguanine			●	●	◎	◎	◎	◎	◎	●			◎	◎		◎				◎				◎	◎
Thiotepa			●	●	●	◎	◎							◎		◎				◎				◎	◎
Topotecan			●	●	◎	◎	◎						◎						◎	◎					
Tretinoin		◎					◎						◎		●					●		◎		◎	
Vinblastine		●	●		◎	◎		●		◎	◎			◎					◎	◎		●	◎		
Vincristine		◎			◎	◎		◎		◎	◎		◎		●	◎		◎	◎	◎					◎
Vendesine		●	◎	◎	◎	◎		◎	◎					●						◎					
Vinorelbine		●	◎	◎	◎	◎				◎				●											◎

GLOSSARY

Adeno:	Prefix meaning glandular.
Adjuvant Chemotherapy:	Chemotherapy used in combination with surgery and/or radiotherapy.
Alkaline Phosphatase:	An enzyme produced in the liver. When the liver is traumatized, it gives off alkaline phosphatase into the blood. It is used as a signature for liver toxicity, which can be due to drugs affecting the liver, cancer in the liver or cancer in the bone.
Alkylating:	Molecules that spontaneously bind to and cross link proteins and DNA. Alkylating agents are a family of drugs used as anti-cancer drugs that work by congealing DNA and the proteins associated with it.
Allogeneic:	Of similar, but not identical genetic background. It is commonly used to describe tissue or organ transplants, where two individuals are similar enough in makeup for one to be able to donate tissue without provoking too serious a rejection reaction.
Alopecia:	Hair loss.
Amenorrhea:	Cessation of menstruation.
Amino acids:	The class of chemical compounds that form the building blocks of polypeptides, proteins and enzymes.
Analgesic:	Pain relieving. Analgesics include mild drugs, like aspirin, acetaminophen, or ibuprofen, as well as narcotic drugs, like codeine or morphine.
Anastomosis:	The interface between two tube like structures, where they join. It can refer to the increase in number of blood vessels that occurs in tumors, or the surgical joining of two sections of bowel.
Anemia:	Abnormally low number of red blood cells.
Antigens:	Molecules, or parts of molecules, that stimulate the activation of the immune system.
Apnea:	Stop breathing.
Apoptosis:	Programmed cell death.
Ascites:	Fluid accumulation in the abdominal cavity.

Autologous:	Self made. In transplantation, when a tissue is readmitted to the same patient, it is an autologous transplant.
Axillary Lymph Nodes:	The cluster of lymph nodes in the arm pit.
Bilateral:	On both sides of the body at once.
Biological Therapy:	Using man-made molecules designed to copy the molecules produced as part of the body's natural defense system.
Biopsy:	A sample of tissue removed for diagnosis.
Bone marrow:	The organ that replenishes blood cells. It is found in most bones, but especially the long bones and the sternum. The marrow fills the hollow cavities within the bones.
Cachexia.	Wasting away, either from disease or malnutrition.
Carcinoma:	Malignant tumors formed from cells of the epithelial tissues. Carcinomas are far more common than sarcomas.
Cardiomyopathy:	Damage to the heart muscle.
Catheter:	A tube inserted in the body, such as the bladder, or into a vein.
Cell:	The simplest autonomous biological unit.
Cell Cycle:	The stages a cell goes through when it reproduces itself.
Centigray:	A unit dose of radiation.
Chemotherapy:	Treatment using chemicals, i.e. drugs. It does not just refer to cancer treatment: antibiotic therapy is also chemotherapy.
Chromosomes:	The package of DNA and proteins that carries the genetic information and divides it between the two cells formed during cell division.
Clavicicular Lymph Nodes:	The lymph nodes found above (superclavicular) and below (subclavicular) the collar bone.
Clinical Trials:	Systematic test of one treatment modality with another under controlled conditions. Clinical trials can also be used to evaluate dietary factors, environmental factors or preventive measures.
Clone:	A cell line that is directly descended from a single cell.
Combined Modality Therapy:	The combination of surgery and/or radiotherapy and/or chemotherapy and/or hormone therapy and/or biological therapy.
Consolidation Chemotherapy:	Chemotherapy that is administered after a relapse has occurred.
Contralateral:	Opposite side.
Creatinine:	A substance given off by the kidneys when they are not functioning normally.

Cyst:	A small vessel, or sac, containing gas or fluid.
Cyto(e):	Cell. As a prefix, e.g. cytobiology is cell biology; as a suffix, e.g. hepatocyte is a liver cell.
Cytoplasm:	The material inside the cell but outside the nucleus.
Debulking:	Reducing the size of a tumor surgically when the entire mass cannot be removed for some reason.
Dehydration:	Water loss. It can be caused by taking in too little fluids or by losing more than is being taken in.
Differentiation:	The process of becoming different. In biology, it refers to the process from which immature cells slowly diverge, such that their descendants will form different organ systems during maturation.
Ductal:	Relating to the ducts that carry milk from the lobules to the nipple.
Dysplasia:	An irregular structure in tissues formed of cells who have lost their awareness of the global architecture in which they are growing.
Dyspnea:	Shortness of breath.
Edema:	Swelling due to accumulation of fluid. The adjective is edematous.
Emesis:	Vomiting.
Enzyme:	A protein or cluster of proteins that catalyzes chemical reactions. Enzymes are active parts of the biological machinery, as opposed to the structural proteins, which are largely passive.
Endocrine:	The system of glands that secrete signal molecules to provoke responses in distant organs to regulate their behavior and coordinate complex reactions.
Epidural:	The encapsulated space just outside the spinal cord.
Epithelium:	A layer of interconnected cells that form sheets which line or cover organs.
Erythrocytes:	Red blood cells. The cells that transport oxygen from your lungs to other organs, and return waste carbon dioxide to the lungs.
Estrogen:	A steroid hormone produced by the ovaries that signals other parts of the body what is needed to support activities going on in the ovaries.
Estrogen Receptor:	The molecule in the receiving cell that accepts the estrogen and translates the signal into a biological response within the cell.
Extravasation:	An event when a needle escapes the vein into which it is inserted, so the injection spills into the surrounding tissue.

	This can cause serious damage to the tissues in the case of certain anti-cancer drugs, like doxorubicin. In rare cases, the damage so severe amputation is necessary.
Fibroblast:	A type of cell found throughout the body that produces or repairs the structural network of fibers in tissues.
Fibrocystic:	Formation of fluid filled cysts in the breast. Often fibrocystic breasts fluctuate with the menstrual cycle.
Fibroids:	A benign tumor made of fibroblasts.
Gene:	A segment of DNA that contains the information to produce one polypeptide. It includes a start sequence, a stop sequence, the information needed to produce the polypeptide, and information for how to process the polypeptide.
Genetic Probe:	A piece of DNA constructed to match a specific sequence in a cell's DNA. Probes bind if the specific sequence is present, and tell us it is there. We can also measure how many copies are present, to find out if a particular sequence has been amplified.
Glucocorticoid:	A family of steroids produced in the cortex of the adrenal gland. When they were first discovered, adrenal steroids were divided into those responsible for salt balance and those that affected sugar digestion. Glucocorticoid is the name give to the latter group of corticosteroids.
Growth Control:	The balance of signals, some stimulating, others depressing, the trigger that induces cells to multiply.
Growth Factor:	A signal that stimulates a cell to multiply.
Hepato-:	Having to do with the liver.
Histo-:	Having to do with tissues.
Hormone:	A chemical signal produced by cells in one organ to signal other organs to change their activities in preparation for some event.
Humoral Immunity:	The part of the immune system that secretes antibodies which circulate to neutralize foreign antigens.
in situ:	Within the original site.
Inguinal:	Relating to the groin.
Invasive cancer:	Cancer that has penetrated the healthy tissues surrounding the site of origin.
Ipsilateral:	Same side.
Leukocyte:	White blood cell. White cells include neutrophils, lymphocytes, monocytes, basophils and eosinophils.
Lobule:	Small lobe or division of a lobe.
Lymph:	The clear, fluid within the lymphatic system.

Lymphatics:	The network of vessels and nodes through which the lymph flows on its way back to the blood system.
Lymphocyte:	A type of leukocyte. B lymphocytes are poised to produce immunoglobulins against foreign antigens. T lymphocytes can be of several types. Helper and suppresser lymphocytes help guide the immune system as to whether it should proceed to build antibodies or not. Killer T cells, as the name suggests, attach to and kill cells to which they have been targeted.
Macrophage:	A mature monocyte that has taken up residence in a tissue to serve as a sentinel, ingesting foreign matter. Virtually every organ contains macrophages, which often are specialized for their rôle in each site.
Malignant:	Capable of invasive growth and metastasis.
Mediastinum:	The trunk of tubes in the center of chest that includes the esophagus, trachea, heart, major blood vessels and surrounding tissues.
Metabolism:	The biological process responsible for synthesis of new biological molecules is called anabolism, and the digestion of large molecules is called catabolism. The whole together, synthesis and breakdown, is termed metabolism.
Metastasis:	Nicknamed "mets." A secondary tumor, formed from a cell that has spread beyond the site of origin. The plural form is metastases. The verb is metastasize.
Mineral-corticoid:	A family of steroids produced in the cortex of the adrenal gland. When they were first discovered, adrenal steroids were divided into those responsible for sugar metabolism and those that affected the proportions of mineral salts in the blood. Mineralocorticoid is the name give to the latter group of corticosteroids.
Mitosis:	The process whereby one cell divides into two daughter cells.
Morbid:	Diseased.
Mucositis:	Inflammation of mucous membranes. Many anti-cancer drugs are toxic to the cells that line the mouth, stomach, and intestines.
Multipotent:	Stem cells that can, when signaled, mature to become more than one end stage cell, depending on the body's needs.
Mutation:	Change or alteration. Specifically, a change in the genetic material (DNA) of cells that is passed on to successive generations of the mutant cell.

Nadir:	Lowest point. For example, it is used to describe the day when your white blood cells are at their lowest, following chemotherapy that causes leukopenia.
Nausea:	The symptoms leading up to vomiting. Feeling sick to your stomach.
Necrosis:	Local zones in a tissue where extensive cell death has caused a disintegration of the structure. Necrotic tissue can heal quickly, or it can become ulcerative and be subject to infection.
Needle biopsy:	A technique for removing a piece of tissue by sucking it into a syringe so it can be tested in a laboratory diagnosis.
Neoadjuvant Therapy:	The technique of reducing tumor size (downsizing) and killing minute tumors in distant sites by treating with chemotherapy prior to surgical resection or radiotherapy.
Neoplasm:	New growth, as in tumor. Refers to both benign and malignant tumors. (the adjective is neoplastic)
Nephro-:	Having to do with the kidneys.
Neutropenia:	Abnormally low numbers of white blood cells, especially neutrophils, circulating in peripheral blood.
Neutrophils:	A type of white blood cell that provides defense against possible invading organisms. Neutrophils are short lived, and, when provoked, throw themselves against a target, releasing highly toxic excretions and sending signals to mobilize other elements of the defense system.
Oncogene:	A piece of genetic material that can turn a normal cell in culture into a cell that becomes malignant. By derivation, it has come to mean a human gene that, when mutated, can establish a malignant tumor.
Oncology:	The field of medicine dealing with cancer.
Oophrectomy:	Surgical removal of the ovaries.
Opportunistic Infection:	An infectious disease that arises because a patients immune system has deteriorated. Bacteria or fungi that ordinarily wouldn't be pathogenic can establish severe, even lethal infections in immune compromised patients.
Palliative:	To remove symptoms, when cure is not possible.
Palpate:	Feel.
Parenteral:	Administration by injection.
Paresthesia:	A burning or tingling sensation, such as you get when you bump your "funny bone."
Petechiae:	Small patches of bleeding under the skin. They are often the first sign of low platelet counts.
Phlebitis:	Inflammation of the veins.

Photosensitivity: Extreme sensitivity to sunlight, such that even a little exposure can cause sunburn.

Platelets: Circulating pieces of cells that, among other things, form blood clots.

Polypeptide: A single polymer of amino acids. It can range in length from a few to hundreds of amino acids long.

Prognosis: Educated guess as to probable outcome.

Prosthesis: An artificial body part, such as a limb or breast.

Protein: An assembly of one or more polypeptides. Proteins are either structural, like collage or silk, or catalytic, as in enzymes, or signals, as in peptide hormones.

Radiotherapy: Treatment using ionizing radiation.

Relapse: Return of a cancer after a period of remission.

Remission: The period during which a disease is undetectable.

Resection: Surgical removal.

Response: Effect of treatment on the tumor. Complete response means elimination of all visible evidence of the tumor. Partial response is defined as tumor shrinkage (of the largest diameter) to less than half what it was before. Stable disease means the tumor stopped growing. No response means just that. N. B. response, even a complete response, does not necessarily mean a cure.

Salvage: An attempt to cure a patient by another type of therapy after a first or second strategy has failed.

Sarcoma: Malignant tumors formed from cells of the connective tissue. These include cancer of the bone and lymphomas.

Staging: Determining the extent of disease and grouping together with patents with similar severity for evaluating treatment options.

Statistics: A branch of mathematics that determines the likelihood of various outcomes in large numbers of trials.

Steroids: A family of molecules that have a characteristic chemical structure for a background upon which are attached one or more side groups. Depending on which side group is attached, different steroids affect a very wide array of cell systems. Study of the interaction of the various steroids and the wide range of affects they promote is a complex and fascinating field.

Estrogen, testosterone, and progesterone are steroids that signal different sexual activities. They trigger activities as diverse as hair growth and lactation. They also give us that peculiar feeling of uneasiness and need for fulfillment that alters our moods and motivates us to aspire for higher things.

Steroids produced in the cortex of the adrenal glands are called corticosteroids. These include mineralosteroids and glucocorticoids. Aldosterone, the primary mineralo-steroid, helps regulate the balance of mineral salts in our blood, and also affects water retention and that feeling of "bloatedness." Glucocorticoids affect protein and sugar digestion. Cortisone and cortisol are other glucocorticoids that suppress control elements in inflammation. They or drugs made to mimic them, are used to control many different inflammatory reactions.

Cholesterol, a major component of all animal cell membranes, is yet another type of steroids.

Stomatitis:	Inflammation of the mucous membranes causing sores or blisters in the mouth. Related to mucositis.
Surgery:	Treatment using mechanical techniques to remove or manipulate the physical components of a system.
^{99}Tc:	A radioactive isotope of the technetium atom that decays very rapidly. It is attached to nutrients that are incorporated into growing cells, to detect tumors growing in metastatic sites, like bone.
Teratogen:	A chemical that causes birth defects.
Thorax:	Chest cavity.
Thrombocytes:	Platelets, which are small pieces of cells that circulate in the bloodstream.
Thrombo-cytopenia:	Deficiency in the number of platelets.
Thrombosis:	Blood clot.
Toxic:	Poisonous.
Tubule:	Small tube.

REFERENCES

[1] It actually takes much longer, because at first, only a handful of patients will be receiving this treatment. When a majority of patients have been treated with the new method, then the number of patients who have lived at least five years will be large enough to affect the overall *statistics*.

[2] Survival statistics include deaths from all causes, not just from cancer, so 100% is impossible.

[3] ASCO (American Society for Clinical Oncology) 1995 Abstract No. 155
Breast Cancer Conservative Treatment: A 2238 Patient Series
Floiras, J.L., Nogues, C, Boudinet, A, Rambert, P, Lasry, S, Tubiana-Hulin, M, Turpin, R, & Rouesse, J

[4] ASCO 1995 Abstract No. 231
A Comparison of Mastectomy with Lumpectomy and Radiation in Stage I and Stage II Breast Cancer Based on Tumor Registry Data
Wooolley, P, LeBlond, V, Antemann, R, Duke, B, Islamoff, I, Schrock, L, Stefanik, D, Stefanick, P, Fikri, E, Furnary, J, Cerimele, N, Max, M, Murali, B, Bush, S, Goldblatt, S, Evans, J, & Yerger, J

[5] The units used to be measured as rads. One cGy equals one rad.

[6] American Society of Clinical Oncology, 435 North Michigan Avenue, Suite 1717, Chicago, Illinois 60611, (312) 644-0828

[7] Cancer Information Service, National Cancer Institute: 1 (800) 422-6237 (Information for Patients) or http://www.nci.nih.gov

[8] ASCO 1995 Abstract No. 116
A Randomized Comparison of Single Agent Induction Chemotherapy v. Standard Chemotherapy for Stage IV Breast Cancer CALGB 8642
Costanza, ME, Henderson, IC, Berry, D, Cirrincione, C, Frei, E, McIntyre, OR, & Weiss, RB

[9] ASCO 1994 Abstract No. 31
Median Survival of 59 Months for Premenopausal Women with ER-Positive Metastatic Breast Cancer, an ECOG Study
Falkson, G, Gelman, RS, Tormey, DC, Falkson, CI, Wolter, JM, Cummings, FJ
Long term survival of 130 premenopausal women with metastatic breast cancer. Accrual completed in 1983. ER positive or unknown women were randomized to oöphrectomy plus chemotherapy vs. chemotherapy alone. ER negative women were given chemotherapy alone. (cyclophosphamide, doxorubicin, 5-FU). No difference was seen between the different treatments. Median survival of 59 months in ER positive women, versus 16.9 months in ER-negative.

[10] ASCO 1994 Education Session
Clinical Decision Making in the Use of Adjuvant Systemic Therapy
Henderson, I. Craig

[11]Lancet 339 p 1-15, 71-85 (1992)
Early Breast Cancer Trials Collaborative Group Systemic Treatment of Early Breast Cancer by Hormonal,
Cytotoxic or Immune Therapy: 1,051 Randomized Trials Involving 32,000 Recurrences and 25,000 Deaths
Among 77,000 women.

[12] ASCO 1995 Abstract No. 106
Impact of Age on Prognosis and Toxicity in Elderly Women with Metastatic Breast Cancer (MBC) Treated
with Tamoxifen (TAM): An Analysis of Patients Entered on Four Prospective Clinical Trials
Dhodapkar, M, Ingle, J, Cha, S, Mailliard, J & Wieand, S
Analyzed 396 postmenopausal women who were involved in four CTs and received TAM as initial therpay
for metastatic disease. Of these 184 were elderly (over 65). Elderly patients fared better than those under 65.
The median time to progression of disease was 10.5 mos for those over 65, but 6.2 months for those 65 and
younger.

[13] J. Clin. Oncol. vol. 11 p 51.
A Dose and Dose Intensity Trial of Cyclophosphamide, Doxorubicin and 5-Fluorouracil As Adjuvant
Treatment of Stage II Node positive Female Breast Cancer
Budman, DR, Wood, W, Henerson, IC, Korzun, AH, Cooper, R, Hart, Ellerton, J, Norton, L, Ferree, C,
Colangelo, A, McIntyre, OR

[14] ASCO 1994 Abstract No. 58
Dose Intensification and Increased Total Dose of Adjuvant Chemotherapy for Breast Cancer: Findings from
NSABP B-22
Dimitrov, N, Anderson , S, Fisher, B, Redmond, C, Wickerham, DL, Pugh, R, Spurr, C, Goodnight, Jr, J,
Abramson, N, Wolter, J C
This was a randomized study of women with positive axillary nodes. All patients received doxorubicin (60
mg/M^2 on days 1, 21,42 and 63). Patients were randomized to standard cyclophosphamide (600 mg/M^2),
dose intensified cyclophosphamide (1.2 gm/M^2 on days 1 and 21) or increased and intensified dosage (1.2
gm/M^2 on days 1, 21, 42 and 63). Survival data not available yet.

[15]ASCO 1994 Abstract No. 59
Tumor Size, Ploidy, S-Phase and ERB-2 Markers in Patients with Node-Negative ER-Positive Tumors:
Findings from NSABP B14.
Costantino, J, Fisher, B, Gunduz, N, Fisher, E, Mamounas, E, Paik, S, Dimitrov, N, Bowman, D, Margolese,
R, Kavanah, M, Shibata, H
There were no differences in survival that correlated with erb B-2 status. Per cent of cells in S phase and
tumour size are good prognostic indicators for disease free survival.

[16]Proc. Amer. Soc. Clin. Oncol. vol 12, p72
erbB-2 (c-erbB-2; HER2-new) and S phase Fraction Predict Response to Adjuvant Chemeotherapy in Patient
s with Node Positive Breast Cancer CALGB Trial 8869
Muss, E, Thor, A, Kute, T, Liu, E, Koerner, F, Berry, D, Cirrincione, C, Budman, D, Wood, W, Barcos, M,
Henderson, IC

[17]ASCO 1994 Abstract No. 68
5 Year Results of a Randomized Comparison of Cyclophosphamide Doxorubicin and 5-FU vs.
cyclophosphamide, methotrexate and 5-FU for node Positive Breast Cancer.
Carpenter, JT, Velez-Garcia, E, Aron, BS, Salter, M, Stahl, Estes, DL, Stagg, N, Bartoluucci, M, Singh, A,
Birmingham, KP.
Southeastern Cancer Study Group. Randomized 528 patients with greater than 1 positive axillary node to
CAF or CMF for 6 cycles. No overall survival difference after 5 years.
CAF = cyclophosphamide 500 mg/M^2, doxorubicin 50 mg/M^2, 5-FU 500 mg/M^2
CMF = cyclophosphamide 600 mg/M^2, methotrexate 40 mg/M^2, 5-FU 600 mg/M^2

[18] ASCO 1994 Abstract No. 50

Cyclophosphamide, Methotrexate, 5-FU versus 5- FU, Epirubicin, Cyclophosphamide Chemotherapy in Premenopausal Women with Node Positive Breast Cancer.
Marty, M, Bliss, JM, Coombes, RC, Wils, J, Amadori, D, Gambrosier, P, Richards, M, Aapro, M, Villar-Grimalt, A, McArdle, C, Woods, E, Coombes, G
International Collaborative Cancer Group. 760 patients randomized to compare CMF to FEC. Each cocktail was tested in two schedules. After 4.5 years, there is no difference between the two cocktails or schedules.
CMF_1 = cyclophosphamide 100 mg/M^2 day 1-14, methotrexate 40 mg/M^2 5-FU 600 mg/M^2 day 1 and 8, repeated every 28 days for 6 cycles
CMF_2 = cyclophosphamide & 5-FU 600 mg/M^2, methotrexate 50 mg/M^2 all on day 1 & 8
FEC_1 = cyclophosphamide & 5-FU 600 mg/M^2, epirubicin 50 mg/M^2 every 21 days for 8 cycles
FEC_2 = cyclophosphamide and 5-FU 600 mg/M^2 days 1 & 8, epirubicin 50 mg/M^2 on day 1 every 28 days for 6 cycles

[19] ASCO 1995 Abstract No. 112
Clinical Trial of Intensive CEF versus CMF in Premenopausal Women with Node Positive Breast Cancer
Levine, M, Bramwell, V, Bowman, D, Norris, B, Findlay, B, Warr, D, Pritchard, K, MacKenzie, R, Robert, J, Arnold, A, Tonkin, K, Shepherd, L, Ottaway, J & Miles, J
Randomized 710 patients to either CEF or CMF treatment arms*. Long term follow up data aren't complete yet, but an interim analysis shows CEF has more side effects, but better survival. 25% of patients in CEF arm have relapsed, while 32% of women in CMF arm have relapsed. Toxicities include febrile neutropenia and acute leukemia.
* Cyclophosphamide (75 mg/M^2) Epirubicin (60) 5-Fluorouracil (500)
Cyclophosphamide (100) Methotrexate (40) 5-Fluorouracil (600)

[20] ASCO 1995 Abstract No. 156
FEC with Epirubicin (50 mg/M^2) Prolongs Time to Progression with respect to CMF Given at Equimyuelosuppressive Doses as Front Line Chemotherapy of Metastatic Breast Cancer
Colajori, E, Ackland, S, Anton, A, Donat, D, Efremidis, A, Ezzat, A, Gerahanovich, M, Kolaric, K, Jassem, J, Lassus, M, Lopez, M, Mickliewics, E, Muse, I, Nagykainai, T, & Porro, M
461 Patients were randomized to either FEC or CMF. The doses and schedules of the two arms were adjusted to be equal in terms of myelosuppressive activity. Patients treated with FEC had a significantly longer time before their disease relapsed and a higher response rate (58%) than CMF (44%). It is too early to evaluate whether there is a survival advantage.

[21] ASCO 1994 Abstract No. 57
Effect of Preoperative Therapy for Breast Cancer on Local-Regional Disease: First Report of NSABP-18
Fisher, B, Rockette, H, Robidoux, A, Margolese, R, Cruz, A, Hoehn, J, Boysen, D, Mamounas, E, Wickerham DL

[22] ASCO 1995 Abstract No. 66
Neoadjuvant Chemotherapy with FNC (Fluorouracil, Mitoxantrone and Cyclophosphamide in Operable Locally Advanced Breast Cancer Allows Breast Conservation
Maltere, P, Martin, M, Piot, M, Manoux, D, Maillart, P, Combe, M, Kamioner, D, Serin, D, Chalmin, B, Renaud, R & Grapin, J
This study used combination chemotherapy to downstage tumors larger than 30 mm prior to resection.
67 Patients with operable local tumors greater than 30 mm entered. 14 CR, 25 PR, 19 Stable disease.

[23] ASCO 1994 Abstract No. 110
The Effectiveness of Follow-up Diagnostic Testing in Patients with Curable Breast Cancer: Results from a Multi-center Randomized Trial
Fossati, R, Apolone, G, Liberati, A, Marsoni, S, Meyerowitz, BE, Mosconi, P, Torri, V

[24] ASCO 1994 Abstract No. 96
Quality of Life with Single Agent Mitoxantrone or Combination Chemotherapy for Advanced Breast Cancer: A Randomized Trial

Simes, FJ, Gebski, V, Coates, AS, Forbes, J, Harvey, V, Van Hazel, G, Tattersall, MHN, Abdi, E, Brigham, B
391 patients randomized to mitoxantrone (14 mg/M^2 i.v. every 21 days) or CMFP (cyclophosphamide 100 mg/M^2 and prednisone 40 mg/M^2 orally on days 1 - 14 with methotrexate 40 mg/M^2 and 5-FU 600 mg/M^2 i.v. on days 1 and 8) cycle repeated every 28 days. Patients were crossed over to the other therapy on the first evidence of failure. Quality of life was assessed every 3 months by 14 linear analogue self-assessment and by clinician using Spitzer index. Response rate for CMFP was 39% vs. 24% for mitoxantrone. There was more toxicity in the CMFP arm (alopecia, mucositis, diarrhea, infection). Overall there was no difference in quality of life between the arms, but the time to first progressive disease was slower for CMFP.

[25] ASCO 1995 Abstract No. 60
Randomized Phase II Trial of Mitoxantrone, 5-FU, and High Dose Leucovorin (NFL) vs Cyclophosphamide, Methotrexaste, 5-FU (CMF) in the First Line Treatment of Metastatic Breast Cancer
Hainsworth, J, Jolivet, J, Hopkins, L & Greco, F
128 Patients with metastatic disease who relapsed after standard therapy were randomly assigned to groups receiving CMF or NFL. Patients treated with CMF, on average, relapsed sooner than those with NFL (13.4 months vs 14.6 months).

[26] ASCO 1994 Abstract No. 63
Dose Intensified Cyclophosphamide/Doxorubicin Followed by Taxol and Adjuvant Systemic Chemotherapy for Node-Positive Breast Cancer (CALGB 9141): Randomized Comparison of Two Dose Levels of G-CSF
Demetri, GF, Berry, D, Younger, J, Robert, NJ, Duggan, D, Stoner, P, Henderson, IC
64 patients have been enrolled in this ongoing study. The purpose is to evaluate the effect of adding Taxol to a dose intensive use of cyclophosphamide/doxorubicin (2 gm/M^2 / 75 mg/M^2 repeated every 3 weeks for 5 cycles) supported with G-CSF followed by taxol (175 mg/M^2 i.v. over 3 hrs repeated every 3 weeks for 4 cycles). Incidence of hospitalization for febrile neutopænia did not differ with the different doses of G-CSF (5 vs. 10 µg/kg). Results are too early to evaluate.

[27] ASCO 1994 Abstract No. 97
Optimal Dose and Sequence Finding Study of Paclitaxel by 3 Hr Infusion Combined with Bolus Doxorubicin in Untreated Metastatic Breast Cancer Patients
Gianni, L, Straneo, M, Capri, G, Villani, F, Munzone, E, Bonadonna, G
15 patients with previously untreated metastatic breast cancer entered. After premedication, taxol was given i.v. in a 3 hr infusion every 21 days. The starting dose (125 mg/M^2)was escalated by 25 mg/M^2 increments until dose limiting toxicity was reached. Bolus doxorubicin was given at 60 mg/M^2 5 min. before of after taxol. The sequence was alternated on different dosings. Doses have been escalated from 125 to 200, and the dose limiting toxicity has not been reached. Toxicities observed include cardiac toxicity in 2 pts after cumulative dose of doxorubicin above 480 mg/M^2. neutropænia, parestesia (burning sensation), myalgia (muscle ache) and mucositis. (Complete Response in 3 patients, Partial Response in 8 patients).

[28] ASCO 1995 Abstract No. 64
Paclitaxel, Mitoxantrone, 5-Fluorouracil, and High Dose Leucovorin (P-NFL) n the Treatment of Metastatic Breast Cancer
Hainsworth, J, Jones, S, Erland, J, Raefsky, E, & Greco, F
32 women with visceral metastases were treated 1 CR, 13 PR, 12 stable disease.

[29] ASCO 1994 Abstract No. 33
Randomized Trial Comparing Zoladex (Goserelin) with Zoladex plus Nolvadex (Tamoxifen) as First Line Treatment for Pre-menopausal Advanced Breast Cancer
Jonat, W, Kaufmann, M, Blamey, RW, Howell, A, Njordenskold, JPB, Forbes, J, Kolvenbag, G
318 premenopausal women with advanced breast cancer were randomized to receive either goserelin alone or goserelin in combination with tamoxifen. Survival data are early, but there is no difference as yet. Time to progression of disease slightly favors the combination.

[30]ASCO 1994 Abstract No. 78

Aredia Infusions in Breast Cancer: A Randomized Phase III Trial to Assess Delay in Progression of Bone Metastases

Latreille, J, Conte, PJ, Mauriac, L, Koliren, L, Ford, JM

295 patients with lytic or mixed lytic/sclerotic bone metastases were randomized to receive chemotherapy alone versus aredia (disodium pamidronate 45 mg *i.v.* over one hour every 3 weeks) plus chemotherapy. Time to progressive disease (as measured by bone scans and x-rays) was 249 days in the aredia + chemotherapy arm versus 168 days in the chemotherapy alone arm. No significant toxicities with aredia.

[31] ASCO 1994 Abstract No. 36

High Dose Epirubicin vs. High Dose Epirubicin + Lonidamine in Advanced Breast Cancer: A Multicenter Randomized Trial

Dogliotti, L, Berruti, A, Buniva, T, Zola, P, Baù, MG, Farris, A, Sarobba, MG, Bottini, A, Arquati, P, Deltetto, F, Gosso, P, Monzeglio, C, Moro, G, Sussio, M, Perroni, D

207 patients with advanced breast cancer who had not received chemotherapy were randomized to receive either epirubicin alone (60 mg/M^2 on days 1, 2) cycle repeated every 21 days, or epirubicin in combination with lonidamine (600 mg/d X os given continuously until administration of epirubicin). Median no of cycles was 6. Better response rate in the combination arm, but no survival data yet.

[32] ASCO 1994 Abstract No. 216

Multicenter, Randomized Trial of *i.v.* Navelbine vs. *i.v.* Alkeran (Melphelan) in Patients with Anthracycline-Refractory Advanced Breast Cancer

Jones, S, Winer, E, Vogel, C, Laufman, L, Barlogie, B, O'Rourke, M, Lembersky, B, Budman, D, Bigley, J, Hohneker, J

179 patients with advanced breast cancer who had failed 1 or 2 previous treatments with chemotherapy with an anthracycline were randomized into one of 2 arms (115 on navelbine, 64 on melphalan). Efficacy measured in response rate and time to disease progression, which favor navelbine. Navelbine was well tolerated, mainly granulocytopænia.

[33] ASCO 1995 Abstract No. 62

US Multicenter Phase II Study of Navelbine and 5 Fluorouracil as First Line Treatment of Patients with Advanced Breast Cancer

Yogel, C, Hochster, H, Blumenreich, M, Davis, H, Graham, M, Fabian, C, Laufman, L, Steinfeldt, H, & Hohneker, J

[34] ASCO 1995 Abstract No. 71

Randomized Comparison of Tamoxifen (TAM) and Two Separate Doses of Toremifene (TOR) in Postmenopausal Patients with Metastatic Breast Cancer

Hayes, D, Van Eyl, J, Hacking, A, Goedhals, L, Bezwoda, W, Mailliard, J, Jones, S, Vogel, C, Berris, R, Shemano, I, & Schoenfelder, J,

648 women ER pos or ER unknown were randomized to receive TAM or TOR (at two dose levels). So far there isn't much difference in response or side effects, except the high dose TOR had increased nausea.

[35] ASCO 1995 Abstract No. 96

Decreased Cardiac Toxicity by TLC D-99 (Liposomal Doxorubicin) in the Treatment of Metastatic Breast Carcinoma (MBC)

Fonseca, GA, Valero, V, Buzdar, A, Walters, R, Wiley, J, Benjamin, R, Ewer, M, Mackay, B, Gordon, D, & Hortobagyi, G

41 patients were treated, and the incidence of heart muscle damage was less than expected, although not eliminated altogether.

[36] ASCO 1995 Abstract No. 61

5-Year Results of High-Dose Sequential (HDS) Adjuvant Chemotherapy in Breast Cancer with more than 10 Positive Nodes

Gianni, A, Siena, S, Bregni, M, Di Nicola, M, Dodero, A, Zambetti, M, Orefice, S, Salvadori, B, Luini, A, Greco, M, Zucali, R, Valagussa, P & Bonadonna, G

67 patients less than 55 years were entered on the study. Course 1 was high dose cyclophosphamide, course 2 was high dose methotrexate with leukovorin rescue, plus vincristine and cisplatin, course 3 was high dose melphalan plus peripheral blood progenitor cell infusion. After the chemotherapy, patients underwent radiation therapy. This is a harsh schedule, and one patient died from the treatment. Two were unable to complete the schedule because of toxicity. Ten patients experienced lung fibrosis due to the radiation. They see 78% overall survival (compared with 60% from CMF/ADM) for patients with more than 10 nodes, and 83% for patients with 10 - 15 nodes (compared with 62%).

[37] ASCO 1994 Education Session
High Dose Consolidation for Stage IV Breast Cancer
Livingston, Robert B.

[38] ASCO 1994 Abstract No 94
High Dose Chemotherapy and Autologous Stem Cell Support in Metastatic Breast Cancer: The University of Chicago Experience
Grad, G, Lane, N, Zimmerman, T, Bitran, J, Mick, R, Williams, S
116 women with metastatic breast cancer were enrolled on one of 3 sequential high dose chemotherapy protocols after having shown either stable disease or response to induction chemotherapy. High dose chemotherapy consisted of cyclophosphamide, thiotepa and BCNU or cyclophosphamide and thiotepa. Patients received either autologous bone marrow support or peripheral blood progenitor cell support. According to survival projections from the available data, high dose chemotherapy achieves durable responses in some women, with the best results in women who achieved a complete response from induction chemotherapy.

[39] ASCO 1995 Abstract No. 148
Hish Dose Chemotherapy with Cyclophosphamide, Thiotepa and Carboplatin & Autologous Bone Marrow Transplant for Patients with Stage II/III Breast Cancer and 10 or Greater Lymph Nodes: Two year Follow-up and Report
Holland, H, Klein, L, Geller, R, Connaghan, D, Devine, S, Dix, S, Fleming, W, Hillyer, C, Miller, R, Morris, L, Winton, E, & Wingard, J
47 patients with Stage II or IIIa breast cancer with 10 or more lymph nodes involved were treated. Treatment consisted of ablative chemotherapy followed by bone marrow transplantation. One patient died due to side effects of the treatment. Two patients have relapsed. The median folow-up is 418 days, and they calculate the two year survival is 87%.

[40] ASCO 1994 Abstract No. 42
Comparative Study of Dose Escalation vs. Interval Reduction to Obtain Dose Intensification of Epirubicin and Cyclophosphamide with GCSF for Patients with Metastatic Breast Cancer
Lalisang, R, Wils, J, Nortier, J, Burghouts, J, Hupperets, P, Erdkamp, F, Schouten, H, Blijham, G (Abstract No. 42)
Phase I/II study. 61 breast cancer patients were randomized to receive either increasing doses of chemotherapy, supported by G-CSF (arm 1) or dose intensification through the use of G-CSF. For arm 1, 5 patients were given a starting dose (epiribicin 140 mg/M^2, cyclophosphamide 700 mg/M^2 that caused 2 toxic deaths. 10 patients received a lower dose (120/700), with 2 episodes of severe toxicity. In arm 2, the interval between chemotherapy treatments (75/500) was shortened from 14 days to 10 days. 8 was deemed improper. Thus G-CSF was more effective in reducing the dose interval than it was for increasing the dose of this combination.

[41] ASCO 1994 Abstract No. 69
Autotransplants for Breast Cancer in North America
Antman, KS, Armitage, JO, Horowitz, MM, Rowlings, PA
Study of 2,500 patients who received autotransplants since 1989. The rapid diffusion of transplant technology has important implications for health care policy.

[42] ASCO 1994 Education Session
Dose Intensive Adjuvant Therapy in Breast Cancer

Antman, Karen H.

[43] ASCO 1995 Abstract No. 67
Combined Modality Approach for Inflammatory Carcinoma of the Breast: 20 Years Experince of M. D. Anderson Cancer Center
Buzdar, A, Hortobagyi, G, Wasaff, B, Holmes, F, Theriault, R Graschini, G, McNeese, M & Singletary, E
MD Anderson treats patients with a combination of radiation, mastectomy and chemotherapy. The chemotherapy consists of FAC* ± vincristine and prednisone. Patients who relapsed after FAC were switched to methotrexate, folinic acid and vinblastine. Altogether, 178 patients have been followed. 27% of patients were free of disease after 15 years.

[44] ASCO 1994 Education Session
High Dose Chemotherapy for Breast Cancer: Efficacy, Cost and Cost-Effectiveness
Smith, Thomas J, Hillmer, Bruce, E., Desch, Christopher E

[45] People familiar with computers may find a better analogy in memory. The DNA is the permanent storage medium, like a hard drive, and the volatile copy (mRNA) is RAM memory. A "byte" of genetic information is called a codon, and a "document" is a gene. A chromosome would be equivalent to a disk partition, or one of a string of hard drives.

[46] ASCO 1995 Education Session
Conceptual Issues in the High Dose Chemotherapy of Breast Cancer
Norton, Larry

[47] To be scientifically accurate, cells do not adapt. Rather, the genetic drift that happens during multiple rounds of replication changes the genes expressed in some cells. For example, all cells have the ability to make the MDR gene product, but most don't. Those that happen to be making it can grow when chemotherapy is given, while those that didn't can't. This may seem a subtle point, but it is important to those who study the mechanisms behind resistance.

INDEX

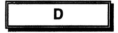
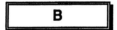
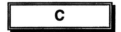
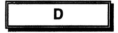
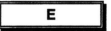

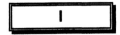
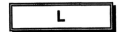

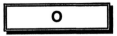
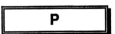

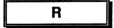
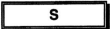
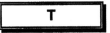